Defeat
MALARIA

Dr Asha Chowdhry

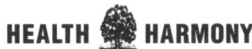

An imprint of
B. Jain Publishers (P) Ltd.
An ISO 9001 : 2000 Certified Company
USA — Europe — India

DEFEAT MALARIA

First Edition: 2010
1st Impression: 2010

All rights reserved. No part of this book may be reproduced, stored in a retrieval system or transmitted, in any form or by any means, mechanical, photocopying, recording or otherwise, without any prior written permission of the publisher.

© with the author

Published by Kuldeep Jain for

HEALTH 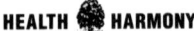 HARMONY

An imprint of

B. JAIN PUBLISHERS (P) LTD.
An ISO 9001 : 2000 certified Company
1921/10, Chuna Mandi, Paharganj, New Delhi 110 055 (INDIA)
Tel.: +91-11-4567 1000 • *Fax:* +91-11-4567 1010
Email: info@bjain.com • *Website:* **www.bjainbooks.com**

Printed in India

ISBN: 978-81-319-0676-7

Dedication

To my father-in-law, Prof. Sher Singh the great academician and a former Union Minister.

Foreword

I deem it my proud privilege to write the foreword to the compilation of 'Defeat Malaria' by Dr Asha Chowdhry. The text is highly relevant, specific and applicable to the programme conditions. The issues/problems raised, priorities indicated in the area of integrated management of the vector borne diseases in India are highly contextual in the successful implementation of the National Vector Borne Diseases Programme (Malaria). Subject of malaria has been dealt with adequately and is very useful to programme managers, teachers and student community persuing professional courses.

The mainstream of AYUSH has also been built within the policy frame as per what the government is propagating it at the PHC, CHC and District level in accordance with the National Health Programme of Malaria.

I congratulate the author for bringing out the excellent compilation on the vital subject of malaria. Hopefully, it gets disseminated widely to defeat malaria.

Dr Sunder Lal
Former Professor and Head of Department,
Department of Community Medicine,
PGIMS, Rohtak (Haryana)

Preface

Why do we Still Need a Book on Defeat Malaria in this Century?

On a rainy day, a young boy about six years old was brought to me. He was shivering with chills and had fainted on the road side.

In my out patient department a pregnant woman comes with a history of second trimester, high fever with chills since last two days. These two incidences made me think that malaria remains one of the most important endemic disease that threats the mankind. The existing, accepted gold standard for diagnosing malaria is the microscopic examination of thick and thin blood smears. This method has the advantage of high sensitivity, quantifiable results, and accurate specification, but is fairly time consuming and requires well trained microscopists in order to detect low parasitemias and to properly differentiate the species. The rapid diagnostic immunocapture test strips do not require the same level of training and equipment as microscopic examination, and are also significantly faster. However, as this review delineates, clinical trials have shown that the strips are not as sensitive as microscopic examination in detecting low level parasitemias, cannot quantify the level of malaria infection and at present, can only differentiate between falciparum and non falciparum malaria. The strips also have problems relating to antigen persistence in the blood after parasite clearance by chemotherapy, leading to false positive post-therapeutic diagnoses.

Acknowledgements

On the very onset I would like to thank Dr Geeta whose *'brain child'* about writing a book on Homeopathic treatment of Malaria was *adopted* by me.

Then it was

'मैं अकेला ही चला था जानिब-ए-मंज़िल मगर, लोग मिलते ही गए और कारवां बनता गया'

(Main Akela Hi Chala Tha Janib-e-Manzil Magar, Log Milte Hi Gaye Aur Karwan Banta Gaya.)

Dr V.K. Chauhan, principal at Dr B.R.Sur Homoeopathic Medical College, Hospital & Research Centre, Moti Bagh, New Delhi not only encouraged me but also supported me morally and academically.

Dr Gulshan Arora, MD (Medicine) and Medical Specialist at Government Hospital, Gurgaon provided me very relevant and all the latest information and data about this *notorious character*. Dr Mayur Jain and Dr Neha Gupta, the interns, extended a helping hand no matter what the time and requirement was.

My family gave me a *'mosquito-net'* like coverage lest this *vector* would have attacked me taking me as its foremost enemy.

Thanks to the publishers who helped me in finishing this *war* quickly.

Can't forget to thank all my friends, colleagues, supporting staff at home and of my college Dr B.R.Sur Homoeopathic Medical College, Hospital & Research Centre, Moti Bagh, New Delhi.

Dr Asha Chowdhry

Publisher's Note

Everybody living in small towns as well as in the big metropolitan cities know just how widespread is the dreaded menace of mosquitoes. One such disease is malaria caused by the ubiquitous parasite, plasmodium. Since the spread of liberalisation and globalisation by the turn of the century, there has been an awakening to the desirability of an enhanced quality of life, and now the role of the individual as well as the community in addition to state efforts in fighting and combating the menace is increasingly being stressed by enlightened sections of the urban elites.

This book by Dr Asha Chowdhry is a timely piece of work which will enrich readers with the basic information regarding malaria, be its causation, symptomatology, prevention and management. It will educate the populace towards inculcation of good habits regarding diet, hygine and cleanliness.

Kuldeep Jain
C.E.O., B. Jain Publishers (P) Ltd.

Contents

Dedication	*iii*
Foreword	*v*
Preface	*vi*
Acknowledgements	*vii*
Publisher's Note	*ix*

CHAPTERS

1. **Introduction** — 1
2. **The Plasmodium Parasite** — 3
   - Biology of the Plasmodium Parasite — 3
   - The Ecology of Malarial Parasite — 12
   - Life Cycle of the Malarial Parasite — 13
3. **The Anopheles Mosquito** — 19
   - Geographical Distribution — 19
   - Biology of Anopheles Mosquito — 19
4. **History and Epidemiology** — 25
   - Origin of Malaria Parasite and its Spread — 25
   - Malaria – Ancient Literature — 29
   - Researchers in the battle against malaria — 32
   - Global Spread of Malaria — 39
   - History of Malaria in India — 41
   - Informative newsy briefs of interest — 46
   - Epidemiology — 54

5.	**Clinical Presentation**	**57**
	• Etiology	57
	• Pathogenesis	59
	• Signs and Symptoms	66
	• Complications	73
	• Differential Diagnosis	76
	• Prognosis	78
6.	**Malaria Associated with Other Diseases**	**81**
	• Malaria in Pregnancy	81
	• Malaria in HIV/AIDS	84
7.	**Investigations**	**93**
	• Routine Laboratory Diagnosis	93
	• Rapid Diagnostic Test	96
	• Elisa Test	97
	• Polymerase Chain Reaction	97
	• Detection of Antimalarial Antibodies	97
	• Intra Leucocytic Malarial Pigment	98
	• Flow cytometry	98
	• Mass Spectrometery	98
8.	**Prevention of Malaria**	**99**
	• Individual Level	99
	• Community Level	102
	• Government Level	102
9.	**Control of Vector**	**107**
	• Strategies for Vector Control	107
	• Vector Control Measures	108
	• Malaria Zones Identification and Management	109
10.	**Travel Precautions**	**111**
	• Risk for Travaellers	112
	• Length of Prophylaxis	116

• Pregnancy and Breastfeeding	120
11. Conventional Treatment of Malaria	**123**
• Drug Resistant Malaria	124
12. Traditional and Complementary Therapies	**127**
• Homeopathy	127
• Herbal Remedies	138
• Ayurveda	139
• Acupuncture	141
• Yoga and Exercises	145
• Juice Therapy	147
• Diet and Nutrition	148
• Home Remedies	149
• Massage	151
• Naturopathy	152
• Aroma Therapy	154
Glossary	*155*
Bibliography	*159*

Chapter 1

Introduction

Malaria is a disease caused by a parasite that is carried from person to person by a mosquito and transmitted by the bite of an infected female, anopheles mosquito. When a female anopheles mosquito ingests blood containing malarial parasites, these parasites reproduce in the mosquito's gastrointestinal tract, and then move to the salivary glands. When this mosquito bites another person, the parasites are injected along with the mosquito's saliva. Inside the human, the parasites move to the liver, where they multiply. The parasites infect red blood cells, multiply inside the red blood cells and eventually cause the infected cells to rupture. Malaria is characterised by extreme exhaustion associated with paroxysms of high fever, sweating, shaking chills and anaemia.

Malaria is endemic in parts of Asia, Africa, Central and South America. It is a protozoan disease caused in humans by four species of the genus Plasmodium namely, P. falciparum, P. vivax, P. ovale and P. malariae.

Identifying the parasite in a blood sample confirms the diagnosis. Blood is taken, smeared onto a slide, stained, and examined under a microscope. More than one sample may be needed to make the diagnosis because the level of parasites in the blood varies over time.

A patient diagnosed with Plasmodium falciparum is an emergency case because the disease affects the brain, heart and kidneys.

Chapter 2

The Plasmodium Parasite

BIOLOGY OF THE PLASMODIUM PARASITE

There are four different types of Plasmodium parasites which cause malaria in human beings.

1. Plasmodium ovale: Causes benign malaria and can stay in your blood and liver for many years without causing symptoms.
2. Plasmodium vivax: Causes benign malaria with less severe symptoms than P. falciparum. P. vivax can stay in your liver for up to three years and can lead to a relapse.
3. Plasmodium malariae: Causes benign malaria and is relatively rare.
4. Plasmodium falciparum: This is the only parasite that causes malignant malaria. It causes the most severe symptoms and results in the most fatalities.

P. falciparum is responsible for about three quarters of reported malaria cases. Most of the other cases of malaria are caused by P. vivax with just a few caused by the other two species. It's possible to get infected with more than one type of Plasmodium parasite. Each parasite causes a slightly different type of illness.

Three factors are essential for the spread of malaria –

1. Agent: There are 60 varieties of Plasmodium but out of them only four types cause malaria and these are Plasmodium falciparum, the cause of malignant malaria, while Plasmodium vivax, Plasmodium ovale and Plasmodium malariae cause more benign types of malaria. Malignant malaria can kill, but the other forms are much less likely to prove fatal. In India 60-65 % cases of malaria are due to P.vivax, and approximately 35-40% are due to P.falciparum.

2. Host: Any one who lives or travels to places which are prone to harbour the anopheles mosquito.

3. Environment: Humid, hot and swampy.

Plasmodium Ovale

Life cycle

The Plasmodium ovale reaches the liver and begins its exo-erythrocytic schizogony stage and merozoites are formed. There are times when some sporozoites do not form merozoites but remain dormant in the hepatocytes for many months and these are known as hypnozoites. These hypnozoites can cause relapse in a person in future. Incubation period is 14 days (16-18 days).

Epidemiology

It is endemic in West Africa, Philippines, Eastern Indonesia and Papua New Guinea.

Symptoms

The symptom onset is like flu and causes benign malaria and can stay in your blood and liver for many years without causing symptoms.

Diagnosis

The microscopic presentation of P.ovale and P.vivax is very much alike and it becomes difficult to isolate them, so it is usually diagnosed as 'P.ovale/vivax'. Since both are a type of benign malaria the treatment remains the same.

Microscopically there are about 20 % of parasitised cells that are oval in shape.

The only differentiating point from P.vivax is that the mature schizont will never have more than 12 nuclei inside the cell.

Microscopically

- Red cells enlarged
- Comet forms common
- Rings large and coarse
- Schuffner's dots, when present, may be prominent

Mature schizonts similar to those of P. malariae but larger and coarser.

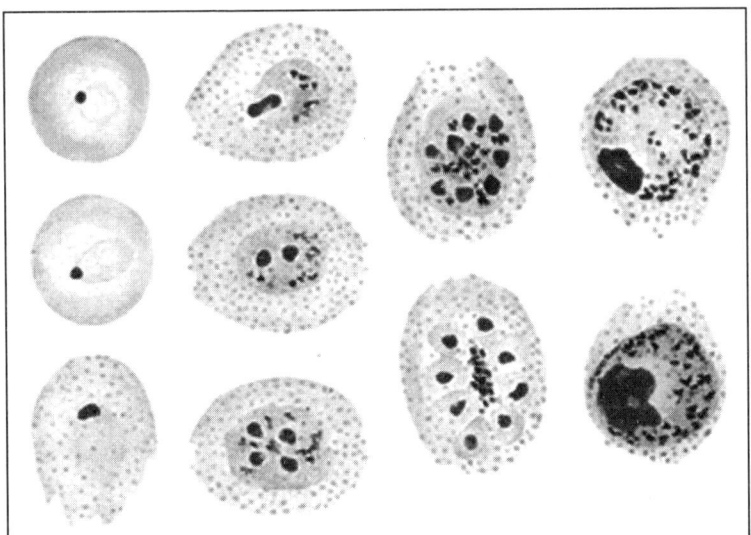

Treatment

Chloroquine and Primaquine.

Plasmodium Vivax

Life cycle

A malaria infected female anopheles mosquito inoculates sporozoites into the human host and these sporozoites infect liver cells and either enter a dormant hypnozoites state or mature into schizonts, which rupture and release merozoites.

The gametocytes are found in the blood at the end of the first week.

Incubation period is 14 days (12-17 days) or may be months.

Epidemiology

Asia, Latin America, some regions of Africa. The most frequent cause of recurrent malaria (Tertian Type). Most people who do not have the antigen against the invasion of red blood cells are resistant to this type of infection.

Symptoms

This causes benign malaria with less severe symptoms than P. falciparum. P. vivax can stay in your liver for up to three years and can lead to a relapse. The infection due to this can be fatal at-times causing marked splenomegaly and then death.

Relapses will occur in 60% of untreated or improperly treated cases.

The blood stage, which requires treatment, is diagnosed by the blood test, which indicates severe anaemia, jaundice and hepatosplenomegaly.

Diagnosis

The P.vivax invades young red blood cells.

The blood film is similar to that of P.ovale and microscopically the parasitised red blood cell is twice the normal size. Schuffner's dots are seen on the surface of the infected cells. The parasite in the cell is irregular in shape and contains 20% merozoites inside the reticulocytes.

Microscopically

- Red cells containing parasites are usually enlarged
- Schuffner's dots are frequently present in the red cells
- The mature ring forms tend to be large and coarse
- Developing forms are frequently present

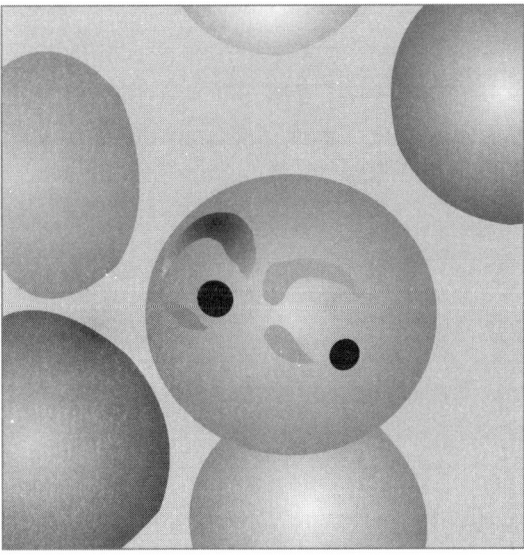

Treatment

Chloroquine is used widely except in Indonesia, Irian Java, Papua

New Guinea where Chloroquine resistance is common. Then mefloquine is given for the treatment.

The most important aspect regarding treatment of P.vivax is that the treatment should be given in respect to the eradication of the liver stage.

Checking the G6PD status and then prescribing Primaquine is also a way to diagnose this.

Plasmodium Malariae

Life cycle

The liver stage has 15 days, and the red blood cell stage is for 72 hours only, hence the fever occurs after 3 days of interval (Quartan Fever).

No persisting hepatic cycle stage hence no relapses.

Epidemiology

This causes malaria in humans and animals both. It is prevalent throughout the world. It is less dangerous than the other 3 varieties of Plasmodium.

Incubation period is 30 days (18-40days).

Symptoms

The prodrome is severe as compared to P.vivax strain and anaemia is less marked.

There is marked splenomegaly but rupture is less prevalent. This can cause infection in the kidneys with poor prognosis.

The parasites can survive in the blood for up to 52 years.

Asymptomatic carriers of P.vivax are diagnosed during the blood donation.

Diagnosis

The parasitised RBC is never enlarged, may appear smaller than normal.

The cytoplasm is normal in colour and no dots are present. The food vacuole is small and parasite is compact. A collection of large grains of parasites, which resembles a band, is characteristic of the P. malariae. The cell has 8 merozoites.

The pathogen P.knowlesi can be mistaken for the P.malariae, so special care is to be taken for accurate diagnosis of the P. malariae.

Microscopically

- Ring forms may have a square in appearance
- Band forms are a characteristic of this species
- Mature schizonts may have a typical daisy head appearance with up to ten merozoites
- Red cells are not enlarged
- Chromatin dot may be on the inner surface of the ring

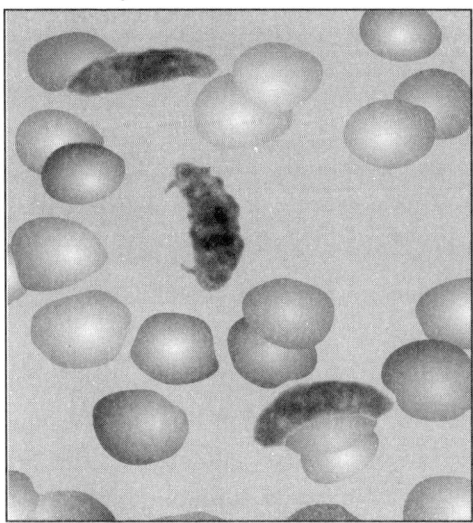

Treatment

Oral Chloroquine is the treatment of choice for uncomplicated Plasmodium malariae infections worldwide.

Plasmodium Falciparum

Life cycle

The female anopheles injects the Plasmodium falciparum and the parasite travels through the blood stream to enter the liver cells or hepatocytes and matures by differentiation into merozoites. After maturation, the merozoites are released from the hepatocytes and enter the erythrocytic stage of their life cycle.

There is no reversion to the hepatocyte.

After entering the erythrocyte the parasite loses its organelles and re-differentiates into a round form in the cytoplasm of the red blood cell (Ring stage).

Epidemiology

Most prevalent in Sub Saharan Africa. Most dangerous of all types, causes malignant type of malaria.

Symptoms

Lacks classical paroxysm and may be followed by an asymptomatic period. Fever is constant or remittent, with headache, muscle pain, and dizziness in postural hypotension.

Jaundice, splenomegaly and cerebral malaria can occur in non-immune patients.

The fever and chill stages of the malaria by P.falciparum are characterised by the timings of rupture of erythrocytic stage schizonts. The parasitised red cells obstruct the capillaries and venules causing local hypoxia and thus releasing toxins. When this affects the arteries of the brain it causes cerebral malaria; the patient can become comatosed and die also, if not treated in time.

Diagnosis

Microscopically

- Rings appear fine and delicate and there may be several in one cell
- Some rings may have two chromatin dots
- Presence of marginal or appliqué forms
- Gametocytes have a characteristic crescent shape appearance
- Maurer's dots may be present
- Red cells are not enlarged

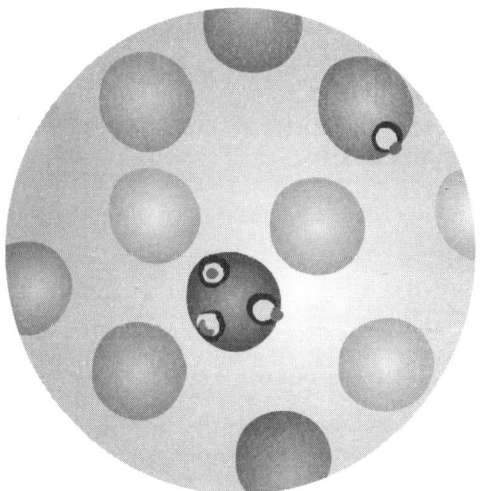

Treatment

Resistance to Chloroquine complicates the treatments of P. falciparum; hence other drugs like Mefloquine, quinine, pyrimethamine/ sulfadoxine (FansidarR), etc., are used.

THE ECOLOGY OF MALARIAL PARASITE

The malarial parasite is a single celled organism, a protozoan. It depends upon female anopheles mosquito to complete its life cycle, maturation and growth.

The female anopheles mosquito injects the sporozoites in the human body where it bites. Man is the only important reservoir.

Vector

Female anopheles mosquito.

Temperature

Maximum of 86°F - minimum of 68°F, it does not survive beyond these temperatures.

Altitude

Rarely exist above 2000 meters.

Terrain and Rainfall

The parasite thrives in heavy rainfall and near the coastal areas and lowlands where they breed.

Transmission

1. Bite of the female mosquito
2. Contaminated needles
3. Blood transfusion
4. Transplantation of the organs
5. Congenital

Susceptibility

Everybody is susceptible to malaria.

Pathogenesis

1. Destruction of the red blood cells
2. Tissue hypoxia
3. Immune complexes and mediators
4. Capillary permeability

LIFE CYCLE OF THE MALARIAL PARASITE

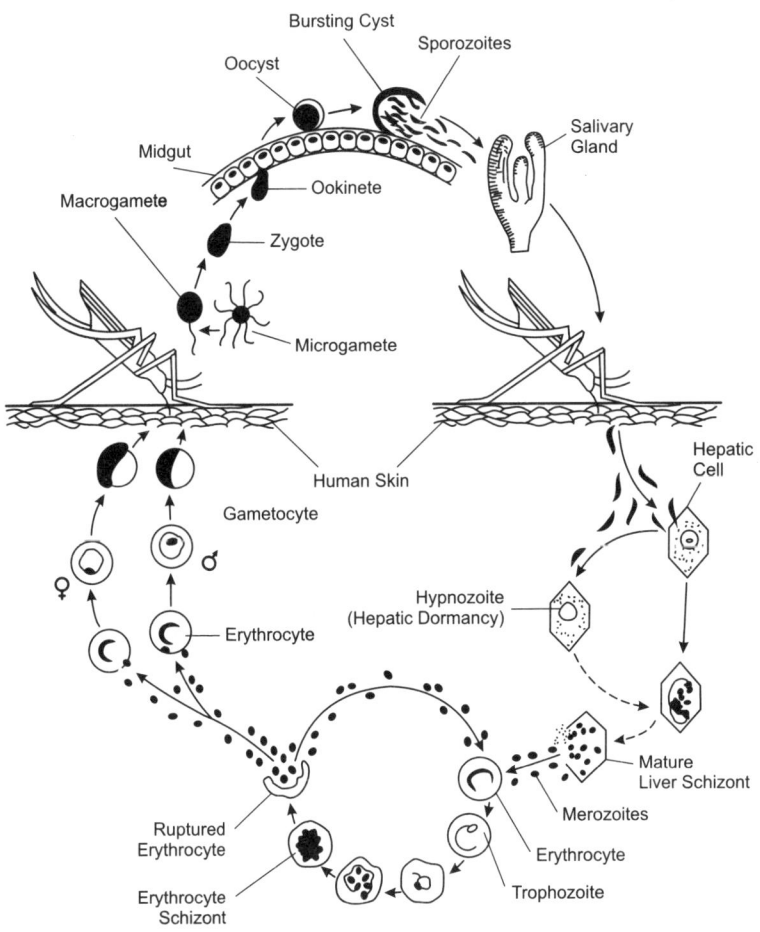

Stage I

The female anopheles mosquito injects the sporozoites in the human body, where it bites and enters the parenchymal cells of liver in 30 minutes after the inoculation.

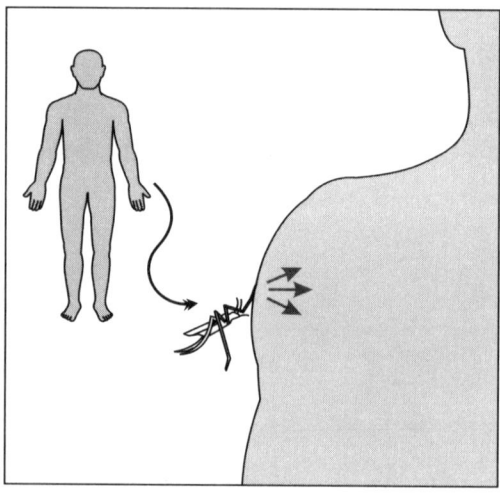

Stage II (Human Liver Stage)

These sporozoites enter the liver cells where they start growing as multinucleated liver stage schizont. This stage stays for 5-21 days.

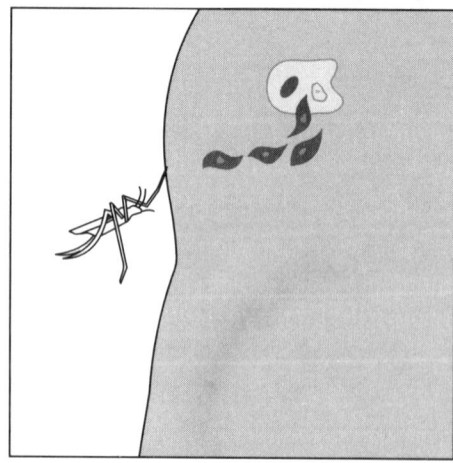

Schizonts rupture and release the merozoites. Over 5-16 days, the sporozoites grow, divide and produce thousands of haploid forms called merozoites. Some malarial parasite species remain dormant for extended periods in the liver, causing relapses weeks or months later.

Stage III (Human Blood Cell Stage)

The merozoites enter the red blood cells, here the fate of these merozoites is either to form the gametocyte or re-enter the blood cells and begin a cycle of invasion of red blood cells, asexual replication and release of newly formed merozoites from the red blood cells repeatedly over 1-3 days. This multiplication can result in thousands of parasite infected cells in the host bloodstream, leading to illness and complications of malaria that can last for months if not treated.

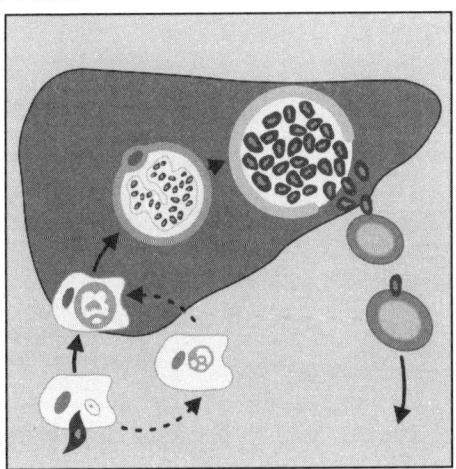

Stage IV (Sexual Stage)

In this stage the gametocytes get differentiated into male and female gametocytes.

Some of the merozoites infected blood cells leave the cycle of asexual multiplication. Instead of replicating, the merozoites in these cells develop into sexual forms of the parasite, called male and female gametocytes that circulate in the bloodstream.

Stage V (Early Mosquito Stage)

At this stage the female anopheles ingests the parasite during her blood meal.

Only the female anopheles needs a blood meal to carry out further development of maturation and reproduction of the parasite.

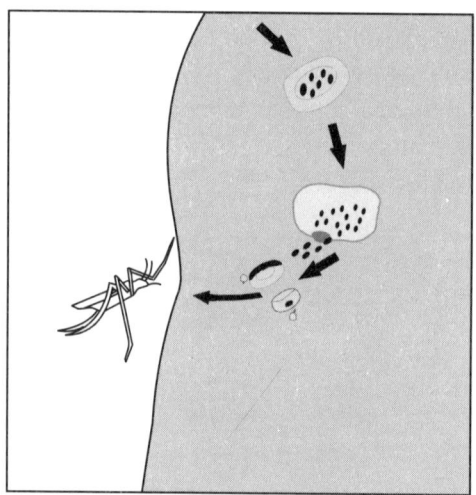

STAGE VI (Intermediate Mosquito Stage)

In this stage the male and female gametocytes unite to form the zygote, which gives rise to ookinete. When a mosquito bites an infected human, it ingests the gametocytes. In the mosquito gut, the infected human blood cells burst, releasing the gametocytes, which develop further into mature sex cells called gametes. Male and female gametes fuse to form diploid zygote, which develop into actively moving ookinete that burrow into the mosquito midgut wall and form oocytes.

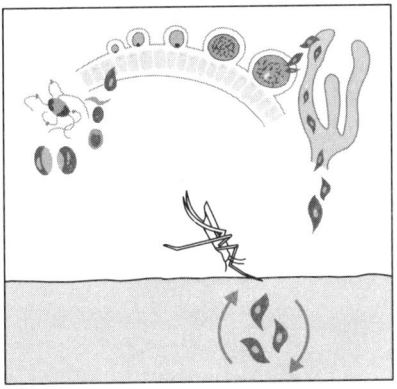

STAGE VII (Late Mosquito Stage)

These Ookinete further grow to form the oocytes, which mature to form the sporozoites.

Growth and division of each oocyst produces thousands of active haploid forms called sporozoites. After 8-15 days, the oocyst bursts, releasing sporozoites into the body cavity of the mosquito, from which they travel to and invade the salivary glands of mosquito. The cycle of human infection re-starts when the mosquito takes a blood meal, injecting the sporozoites from its salivary glands into the human bloodstream.

And again…STAGE I

Chapter 3

The Anopheles Mosquito

GEOGRAPHICAL DISTRIBUTION

Geographical distribution of mosquito vector anopheles in the world: Afro-Arabian areas.

BIOLOGY OF ANOPHELES MOSQUITO

Out of 3,500 species of mosquitoes and out of them only the female anopheles transmits the malaria in human beings.

Life Stages

Eggs, larvae, pupae and adult stage.

The first three stages require water as the medium for growth. This stage lasts for about a fortnight. The adult stage begins when the female anopheles becomes a vector to malaria. The life of an adult female is 1-2 weeks in nature.

Eggs

Adult females lay 50-200 eggs per oviposition, singly and directly on water. They are unique in having floats on either side. Eggs

Eggs

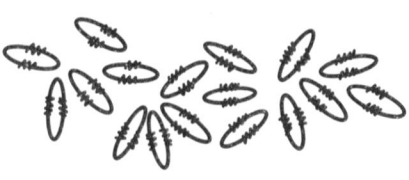

are not resistant to drying and hatch within 2-3 days, in colder climates hatching may take up to 2-3 weeks.

Larvae

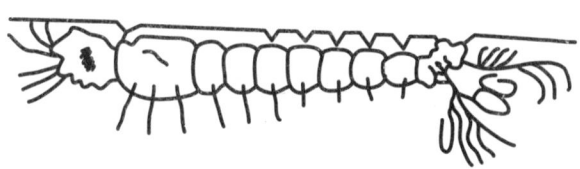

Structures

1. A well developed head with mouth brushes used for feeding.
2. A large thorax and a segmented abdomen.
3. They have no legs and no respiratory siphon.
4. Their bodies are parallel to the surface of the water.
5. Larvae breathe through spiracles located on the 8th abdominal segment.
6. The bodies are placed parallel to the surface of the water for breathing.

Feeding

The larvae feed on algae, bacteria, and other microorganisms.

Movement

Larvae swim either by jerky movements of the entire body or

through propulsion with the mouth brushes, and dive under water when disturbed by external forces.

Habitats

1. Prefer clean, unpolluted water.
2. In fresh or salt water marshes, mangrove swamps, rice fields, grassy ditches, the edges of streams and rivers, small and temporary rain pools.
3. Many species prefer vegetations and some prefer ground without any vegetation around.
4. Some breed in open, sun-lit pools or in shaded breeding sites in forests.
5. A few species breed in tree holes or the leaf axils of some plants.

Larvae develop through 4 stages, they shed their exoskeletons for further growth into the formation of pupae.

Pupae

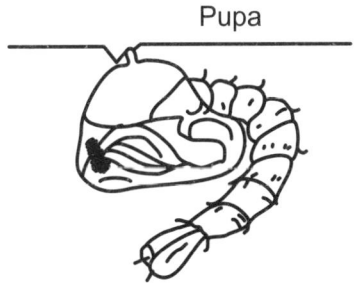

Pupa

Comma shaped. Head and thorax are merged together called as cephalothorax, which have a pair of respiratory trumpets for breathing.

The abdomen is curved underneath.

After a few days as a pupa, the dorsal surface of the cephalothorax splits and the adult mosquito emerges.

Adults

Structure: head, thorax and abdomen.

- **Head**

    Features: A pair of eyes and a pair of long, many segmented antennae, proboscis.

    Function: For acquiring sensory information and for feeding.

    The antennae are important for detecting host odours as well as odours of breeding sites where females lay eggs.

- **Thorax**

    Features: Have three pairs of legs and a pair of wings which are attached to the thorax.

    Function: For locomotion.

- **Abdomen**

    Features: A belly.

    Function: For the digestion of food and development of the eggs.

    When a female anopheles takes a blood meal, the blood acts as a source of protein for the production of eggs and takes a sugar meal for energy.

1. P.ovale: Infects young red blood cells and it has a liver phase.

2. P.vivax: This also infects young red blood cells and it has a liver phase.

    30-40% of malarial cases are due to this species.

3. P.malariae: This infects older red blood cells, so this can persist in the person sub clinically for a very long period.

4. P. falciparum: This infects all the stages of red blood cells, young till old.

   40-60 % of cases are due to this species.

   Most severe and prevalent of all the species.

Incubation Periods of all the Species

P.ovale: 14 days (16-18 days)

P.vivax: 14 days (12-17 days) or months

P.malariae: 30 days (18-40 days)

P.falciparum: 12 days (9-14 days)

   Yet some strains may survive in the humans even for months and years.

Chapter 4

History and Epidemiology

Malaria is endemic in parts of Asia, Africa, Central and South America. It is a protozoan disease caused in humans by four species of the genus Plasmodium namely, P. falciparum, P. vivax, P. ovale, and P. malariae.

Identifying the parasite in a blood sample confirms the diagnosis. Blood is taken, smeared onto a slide, stained, and examined under a microscope. More than one sample may be needed to make the diagnosis because the level of parasites in the blood varies over time.

A patient diagnosed with plasmodium falciparum is an emergency because the disease affects brain, heart and kidneys. Malaria is an infectious disease and as soon as the patient is diagnosed it should be notified immediately.

ORIGIN OF MALARIA PARASITE AND ITS SPREAD

Malarial parasites have been with us since the origin of mankind. They probably originated in Africa. Fossils of mosquitoes up to 30 million years old, show that the malaria vector, the anopheles mosquito, was present well before the earliest history. Hippocrates, a physician in ancient Greece 'Father of Medicine' was the first to describe the manifestations of the disease and related them to the time of year and to where the patients lived. The association with stagnant waters (breeding grounds for the anopheles mosquito) led the Romans to begin drainage programs, the first intervention against malaria.

Malaria has been responsible for the decline of nation's resources and crushing military defeats, often having caused more casualties than the weapons themselves. For centuries it prevented any economic development in vast regions of the earth. It continues to be a huge social, economical and health problem, particularly in the tropical countries.

The most, if not all, of today's population of human malaria had their origin in West Africa (P. falciparum) and West and Central Africa (P. vivax) on the basis of the presence of homozygous alleles for haemoglobin C and RBC Duffy negativity that confer protection against P. falciparum and P. vivax respectively.

Ancestors of the malarial parasites have existed for at least half a billion years. Molecular genetic evidence strongly suggests that the pre-parasitic ancestor for malarial parasite was a chloroplast containing, free living protozoan, which became adapted to live in the gut of a group of aquatic invertebrates. This single celled organism probably had obligate sexual reproduction, within the mid gut lumen of a host species. At some point of time relatively in the early stage of their evolution, these 'pre-malaria parasites' acquired an asexual, intracellular form of reproduction called schizogony, which greatly increased their proliferative potential (schizogony in the RBCs causes the clinical symptoms of malaria).

Among the invertebrates to which the ancestors of the malaria parasites became adapted were probably aquatic insect larvae, early Dipterans (150 to 200 million years ago). During or following this period, certain lines of the ancestral malaria parasites achieved two host life cycles which were adapted to the blood feeding habits of the insect hosts. The malaria parasites infecting humans evolved on this line with alternate cycles between humans and the blood feeding female anopheles mosquito hosts. Fossil mosquitoes have been found in geological strata 30 million years old.

P. malariae, P. ovale and P. vivax diverged over 100 million years ago along the lineage of the mammalian malaria parasites. P. ovale is the sole known surviving representative of its line and causes infection only in humans. P. malariae was a parasite of the ancestor of both humans and African great apes and had the ability to parasitise and cross infect both host lineages as they diverged around five million years ago. P. malariae is found as a natural parasite of chimpanzees in West Africa and P. brazilianum that infects new world monkeys in Central and South America is morphologically indistinguishable from P. malariae. P. malariae, like P. ovale, is the only confirmed and extant representative of its line. P. vivax belongs to a group of malaria parasites like P. cynomolgi, that infect monkeys. The time of divergence of P. vivax from P. cynomolgi is put at 2-3 million years ago.

End of the last glacial period and warmer global climate heralded the beginnings of agriculture about 10,000 years ago. It is argued that the entry of agricultural practice into Africa was pivotal to the subsequent evolution and history of human malaria. The Neolithic agrarian revolution, which is believed to have begun about 8,000 years ago in the 'Fertile Crescent,' southern Turkey and north-eastern Iraq, reached western and central Africa around 4,000 to 5,000 years ago. This led to the adaptations in the anophele vectors of human malaria.

At this time human populations changed from a low density mobile hunting and gathering lifestyle to communal living in settlements cleared in the tropical forest. This new, man made environment led to an increase in the number and density of humans on the one hand and generated numerous small water collections close to the human habitations on the other. Henceforth the increase in the mosquito population was noticed, leading to very high anthropophily and great efficiency of the vectors of African malaria. Even though the practice of agriculture had developed throughout the tropics and subtropics of Asia and the Middle East up to several thousand years before those in Africa, simultaneous animal domestication in Asia probably prevented the mosquitoes from developing exclusive anthropophilic habits. In most parts of the world, the anthropophilic index (the probability of a blood meal being on a human) of the vectors of malaria is much less than 50% and often less than 10 to 20%, but in Sub-Saharan Africa, it is 80 to almost 100%. This is probably the most important single factor responsible for the stability and intensity of malaria transmission in tropical Africa today.

Malaria – Time Frame (Discoveries)

Time Line For Origin of Malaria
Half a billion years ago Existence of pre-parasitic ancestor
150 million to 200 million years ago Early Dipterans, ancestors of mosquitoes appear
130 million years ago Two host life cycle in Dipterans and vertebrates evolves
130 million years ago Divergence of the bird and mammalian malaria parasites
100 million years ago Lineage of P. malariae, P. ovale, and P. vivax diverges
~5 million years ago P. falciparum evolves

2-3 million years ago Divergence of P. vivax from P. cynomolgi
4000-10000 years ago Lethal strain of P. falciparum appears
4000-5000 years ago Anopheles in Africa develop highly anthropophilic habits

MALARIA – ANCIENT LITERATURE

Malaria can be found in the ancient Roman, Chinese, Indian and Egyptian manuscripts and later in numerous Shakespearean plays. The belief that mosquitoes transmit disease also is an ancient one.

One of the oldest scripts, written several thousand years ago in cuneiform script on clay tablets, attributes malaria to Nergal, the Babylonian god of destruction and pestilence, pictured as a double winged, mosquito like insect. A few centuries later, the natives told Philistines settling in Canaan, on the eastern shore of the Mediterranean, of the god Beezlebub, lord of the insects. The evil reputation of this deity increased through the ages until the early Jews named him 'Prince of the Devils.'

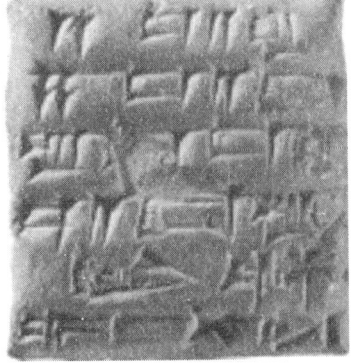

The connection between malaria and swamps was known even in antiquity and the evil spirits or malaria gods were believed to live within the marshes. This belief is likely the origin of the Greek fable of Hercules and Hydra.

The chinese *Nei Ching* (The Canon of Medicine), dated 4,700 years ago, apparently refers to repeated paroxysmal fever associated with enlarged spleen and a tendency to epidemic occurrence, suggesting P. vivax and P. malariae infections.

Sumerian and Egyptian texts dating from 3,500 to 4,000 years ago refers to fever and splenomegaly, suggestive of malaria. The Sumerian records apparently make frequent reference to deadly epidemic fevers, probably due to P. falciparum.

The Vedic (3,500 to 2,800 years ago) and Brahmanic (2,800 to 1,900 years ago) scriptures of Northern India (Indus valley) contain many references to fevers akin to malaria. They are also said to make reference to autumnal fevers as the 'King of diseases'. The *Atharva Veda* specifically details the fact that fevers were particularly common after excessive rains (mahavarsha) or when there was a great deal of grass cover (mujavanta). The ancient Hindus were also aware of the mosquito's harmful potential. In 800 B.C. the sage Dhanvantari wrote, 'Their bite is as painful as that of the serpents and causes diseases... The wound as if burnt with caustic or fire, is red, yellow, white and pink in colour, accompanied by fever, pain of limbs, hair standing on end, vomiting, diarrhoea, thirst, heat, giddiness, yawning, shivering, hiccups, burning sensation, intense cold...' *Charaka Samhita*, one of the ancient Indian texts on Ayurvedic medicine which was written in approximately 300 B.C., and the *Susruta Samhita*, written around 100 B.C., refers to diseases where fever is the main symptom. The Charaka Samhita classifies the fevers into five different categories, namely continuous fevers (*samatah*), remittent fevers (*satatah*), quotidian fevers (*anyedyuskah*), tertian fevers (*trtiyakah*) and quartan fevers (*caturthakah*) and *Susruta Samhita* even associated fevers with the bite of the insects.

Malaria appeared in the writings of the Greeks from around 500 B.C. Hippocrates, 'The Father of Medicine' and probably the first malariologist, described the various malaria fevers of man by 400 B.C. Hippocratic corpus distinguished the intermittent malarial fever from the continuous fever of other infectious diseases, and also noted the daily, every-other-day, and every-third-day temperature rise. The Hippocratic corpus was the first document to mention about splenic change in malaria and also it attributed malaria to ingestion of stagnant water: 'Those who drink (stagnant water) have always large, stiff spleens and hard, thin, hot stomachs, while their shoulders, collarbones, and faces are emaciated; the fact is that their flesh dissolves to feed the spleen...' Hippocrates also related the fever to the time of the year and to where the patients lived.

The recurrence of malaria is a phenomenon that was known to the ancients and first recorded by Roman poet Horace (December 8, 65 B.C. - November 27, 8 B.C.) in his third satire.

In the era of Pericles, there were extensive references to malaria in the literature and depopulation of rural areas was recorded. By about 30 A.D., Celsus described two types of tertian fevers and agreed with the views expressed by Varro. 150 years later, Galen, a famed and influential physician in Rome, recognised the appearance of these fevers with the summer season and jaundice in infected people. But he believed that malaria was due to a disorder in the four humors of the body. According to him, tertian fever was the result of an imbalance of yellow bile; quartan was caused by too much black bile, quotidian by an excess of phlegm and a blood abnormality was the cause of continuous fever. Galen suggested that the normal humoral balance should be restored by bleeding, purging or even better, by both. These tenets were accepted without question for the next fifteen hundred years.

Dante [1265-1321] wrote this on malaria: 'As one who has the shivering of the quartan so near,/ that he has his nails already pale/ and trembles all, still keeping the shade,/ such I became when those words were uttered.' (The Inferno) He died of malaria.

Artist Albrecht Dürer, who contracted malaria in 1520 during a trip to the province of Zeeland in Holland, sought medical advice by sending his physician a sketch showing the upper half of the his body, with an index finger pointing to a yellow spot over the spleen, noting that he felt hurt over that area.

William Shakespeare (1564–1616), mentioned *ague* (English word for malaria) in eight of his plays.

RESEARCHERS IN THE BATTLE AGAINST MALARIA

Malaria has caused much pain and suffering, and for this reason it has attracted since antiquity, some of history's most enquiring minds.

One of the oldest references to this killer disease is preserved in the clay tablets, from Babylon. On these is recorded in the cuneiform script, the cause of malaria as being Nergal. This god of destruction and pestilence is pictured as a double winged, mosquito like insect.

In 800 B.C. the Indian tradition has it that the sage Dhanvantari wrote that the mosquito bites could cause fever and shivering. In 300 B.C. an ancient treatise, the 'Charaka Samhita', classified the fevers into five types, continuous, remittent, tertian, quotidian and quartan fever. Another work, the 'Susruta Samhita', written around 100 B.C. associated some fevers with insect bites.

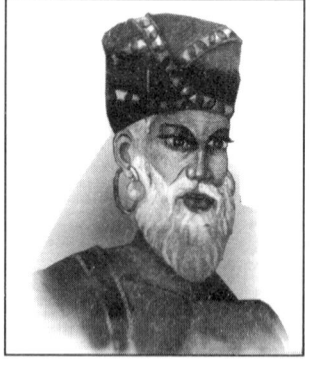

However, it was ancient Greece which produced Hippocrates and he is venerated as the 'Father of Medicine', whose oath, the Hippocratic oath, was for centuries an obligation that each doctor was bound to observe. He is also revered as the first malariologist. The 'Hippocratic Corpus' was the first document to record splenic changes in malaria and how stagnant and still water caused malaria when ingested. The corpus records: 'Those who drink (stagnant water) have always large, stiff spleens and hard, thin, hot stomachs, while their shoulders, face and collar bones are emaciated; the fact is that their flesh

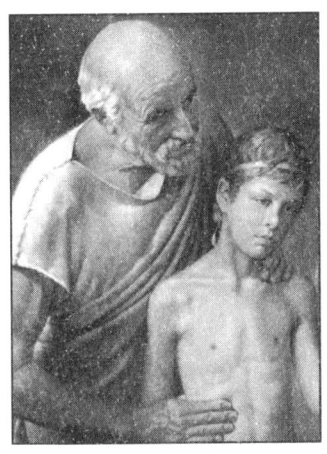

dissolves to feed the spleen.... Hippocrates also related the fever to the season and the surroundings where the patients lived.

In the first century A.D., Roman Scholar Marcus Terentius Varro (116-27 BC) suggested that swamps breed 'certain animalcula which is invisible to the eye and which we breathe through the nose and mouth into the body, where they cause grave maladies'.

Celsus in 30 A.D. concurred with Varro's views and described two types of tertian fevers.

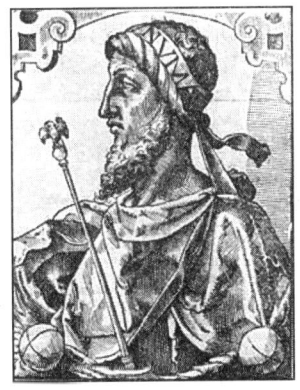

However, these useful observations were subverted by Galen's Dogmatic that theorised that the cause of malaria was internal and this appeared to be widely accepted. Thus, scientific progress was impeded for centuries.

Clandius Galenus of Pergamum (131-201 A.D.) believed that malaria was caused by a disorder in the four humors of the body. His tenets were accepted uncritically for the next 15 centuries. According to him, tertian fever was the result of an imbalance in yellow bile, quartan was caused by too much black bile, and quotidian by an excess of phlegm and a blood abnormality was the cause of malarial fever. Galen suggested that the normal humoral homeostatis should be restored by bleeding, purging or both. The vomiting accompanying malaria was believed by him to be the 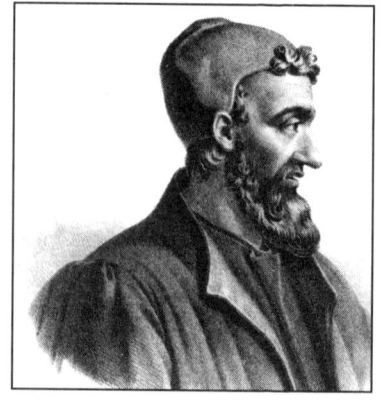 body's bid to eject poisons. The bleeding possibly rid the body of 'corrupt humors'. With the renaissance and the enlightenment in Italy there was much surer enquiry into the malady of malaria. Italian physician Giovanni Maria Lancisi in 1716, first described a characteristic black pigmentation of the brain and the spleen

in malaria patients. Lancisi found stagnant water or swamps and their poisonous vapours linked to malaria. On the role of mosquitoes in spreading the disease, he had two postulates. One that the insects deposit micro organisms in uncovered food and drinks and when humans ate this contaminated material, they got malaria. Lancisi's second postulate was more accurate.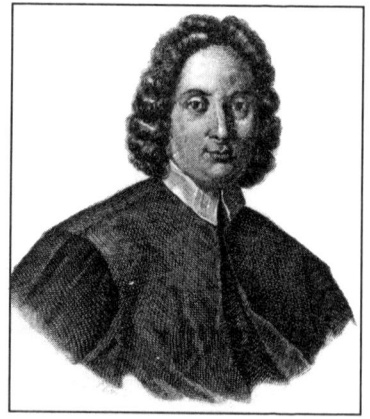

He wrote, 'mosquitoes always inject their salivary juices into the small wounds which are opened by the insects on the surface of the body'.

In 1816, another Italian, Giovanni Rasori (1766-1837) of Parma, while suffering from malaria fever in prison, doubted the 'noxious vapours theory' and suggested that a micro organism was the cause of the disease. He theorised that a parasitical insect caused the paroxysms and intermittent fevers of malaria.

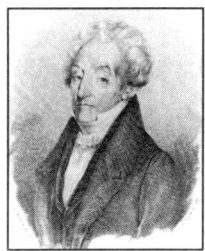

As the 19th century progressed, so did the scientific investigation into malaria and its etiology. In 1850 in his essay 'Yellow Fever Contrasted with Bilious Fever', an American, Josiah Clark Nott, argued that microscopic 'insects' somehow transmitted by mosquitoes caused both malaria and yellow fever. In 1854, another American, Lewis Daniel Beauperthy wrote that marshes, swamps and other stagnant pools were not treacherous because of the miasmic vapours which emanated from them but by the mosquitoes which breeded in them.

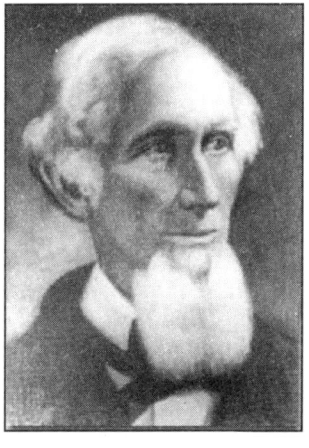

By 1878-79 research into malaria went awry and completely off the track of truth. Under the spell binding germ theory of disease when all epidemic diseases were sought to be blamed on bacteria, an announcement was greeted with wide excitement, 'malaria bacillus' had been found. There was very little skepticism. Edwin Klebs, the German pathologist who had isolated the diphtheria bacillus and Corrado Tommasi-crudeli, an Italian bacteriologist, isolated a microbe from the soil, a short rod that they termed Bacillus malariae, in Roman Campagna.

By 1881, it was shown positively that the Bacillus malariae of Klebs and Tommasi-crudeli was not responsible for malaria. A

U.S. Army major, a bacteriologist of high standing, by the name of George Sternberg, had been sent to new Orleans to study the high incidence of malaria there. He made bacterial cultures from mud, from the marshes and from the air and no organism he found was capable of producing malaria in an animal.

In 1888, a student of Pasteur Alphonse Laveran, a French physician in Algeria, identified the malaria parasite. He named the living organism which was identified on Nov 6, 1880 while he was examining fresh blood specimen taken from a new hospital arrival as 'Oscillaria malariae'. A moving object on the slide caught Leveran's eye. Under high power, this proved 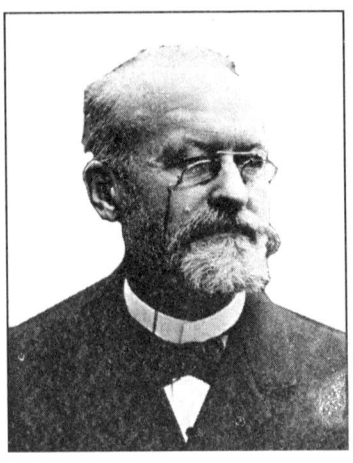 to be a tiny malarial body wriggling vigorously. He immediately realised, as he watched amazed, that he had found a living organism that caused malaria. His observations were quickly confirmed by the Academy of Medicine in Paris. In 1907, he was awarded the Nobel Prize for medicine and the citation read, 'In recognition of his work on the role played by protozoa in causing diseases'.

Laveran's theory was challenged by Dr William Osler an authority on blood microscopy. In 1886, he stated that the malarial bodies were nothing more than incidental findings. Upon being urged by his colleague to reconsider, he, after much study, confirmed Laveran's findings with his own description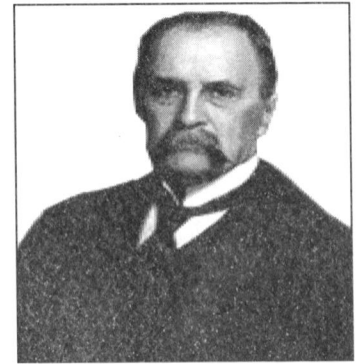

of blood film examinations from 70 patients. Osler also instituted routine blood smear analysis to diagnose malaria in the work-up of febrile patients at Johns Hopkins hospital. In the first edition of his great textbook, 'The principles and practice of medicine', in 1892, Osler continued to maintain a peculiar ambivalence towards the cause of malaria.

In 1885, Camillo Golgi, an Italian neurophysiologist, established that there were at least two forms of the disease, one with tertian periodicity (fever every other day) and one with quartan periodicity (fever every third day).

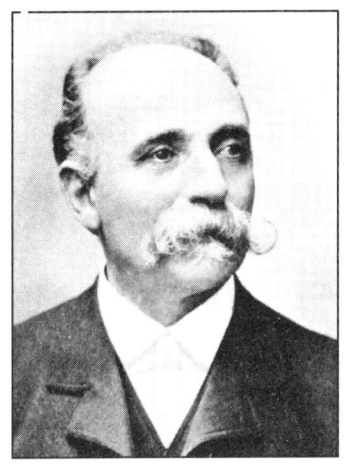

In 1886, he was the first to observe that tertian and quartan forms produce different number of segmentations on maturity, implying that the two diseases were caused by two distinct parasites. He also showed that the fever coincided with the rupture and release of merozoites into the blood stream and that the severity of symptoms correlated with the number of parasites in the blood. In 1906, he was awarded the Nobel Prize in medicine for his path breaking discoveries in neurophysiology.

Patrick Manson while working in China also engaged in the study and reflection on the nature of malaria. He sought to compare malaria with filariasis, for which the mode of transmission by mosquitoes was discovered by him. In Scotland, he could finally get to see Laveran's malarial parasite and he studied the

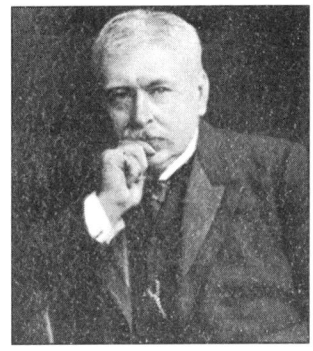

observations of Laveran, Golgi and others. He then confirmed to his own satisfaction that there were several types of parasites that could infect a human being, each having its own appearance and producing its own signs and symptoms.

Ronald Ross was a reluctant physician in the Indian medical service with an incredibly ambitious mindset. He had hoped to write soul stirring poetry, compose music, be a playwright and novelist and revolutionise maths. Instead, he was stimulated by Manson into research and testing of Laveran and Manson's mosquito theory. By the late 1890s the mosquito hypothesis could be established. Ross set out on 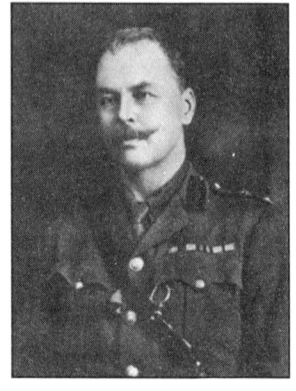 his long and arduous journey of research without a reading of the masters and earlier experts. Still, he came to know most of the things independently. During his work in many hospitals in India, Ross studied mosquitoes in great and minute details and studied their habits and habitats besides finding in them the vector for malaria. His single minded body of work laid the foundations of and paved the way for later malaria control efforts. Ross's discoveries into malaria were immediately followed by a series of important works by Grassi, Robert Koch and others which made valuable contributions in combating and preventing the malaria disease, enlarging the man's understanding of malaria in a wide spectrum.

In 1973, human protection from malaria by vaccination was first reported. For about 20 years, progress occurred mainly in experimental models rather than in human vaccine trials. In 1987, Dr Mannel Elkin Pat arroyo, a Colombian biochemist, developed the first synthetic Spf 66 vaccine against P. falciparum parasite. During the last 5 years or so, many candidate vaccine approaches have been tested in clinical trials. Newer diagnostic tests have been developed for malaria.

GLOBAL SPREAD OF MALARIA

With the origin in the West and Central Africa, malaria spread all across the globe. The parasites spread to other areas through the journey of man, following the human migrations to the Mediterranean, Mesopotamia, the Indian Peninsula and South-East Asia. Men from ancient China almost 5000 years ago, who travelled to malarious areas were advised to arrange for their wives to be remarried. Sumerian and Egyptian texts dating from 3,500 to 4,000 years ago mention about fevers and splenomegaly suggestive of malaria (the enlarged spleens of Egyptian mummies are believed to have been caused by malaria). It appears that P. falciparum had reached India by around 3,000 years ago. It is believed that malaria reached the shores of the Mediterranean Sea between 2,500 and 2,000 years ago and northern Europe probably between 1,000 and 500 years ago.

The waves of invasions that swept across the continents helped the cause of malaria parasite as well. By the Middle Ages, Kings and feudal lords had the best wetlands under their control, but in turn had to fear marshes as breeding grounds of plagues and incurable fevers. A royal decree was passed in 11th century Valencia sentencing any farmer to death who planted rice too close to villages and towns and the conflict between rice growers and the authorities continued for centuries. The disease continued its spread and decimated local populations with the increase in rice farming.

By the beginning of the Christian era, malaria was widespread around the shores of the Mediterranean, in southern Europe, across the Arabian peninsula and in Central, South and South-East Asia, China, Manchuria, Korea, and Japan. Malaria probably began to spread into northern Europe in the Dark and Middle Ages via France and Britain. The growth in international trade in the sixteenth century contributed to the spread of disease, as international traders introduced new sources of infection. Europeans and West Africans introduced malaria in the New World at the end of 15th century A.D. P. vivax and P. malariae were possibly brought to the New World from South-East Asia by early trans Pacific voyages.

P. falciparum probably reached America through the African slaves brought by the Spanish colonisers of Central America. Over the next 100 years, malaria spread across the United States of America and Canada and by around 1850 A.D., it prevailed through the length and breadth of the two American continents. At this time, malaria was common in Italy, Greece, London, Versailles, Paris, Washington D.C. and even New York City.

Thus by 19th century, malaria reached its global limits with over one half of the world's population at significant risk and 1 in 10 affected expected to die from it. From the mid 19th century onwards, with the use of the Cinchona bark, mortality rates fell rapidly to less than one quarter of this. Up to early 20th century, repeated untreated infections of P. vivax and prolonged infections of P. malariae also contributed significantly to the mortality along with the lethal P. falciparum.

Poor living conditions, poverty and famine probably contributed to the high mortality. During the past 100 years, nearly 150 million to 300 million people would have died from the effects of malaria, accounting for 2-5% of all deaths. In the early part of the century, malaria probably accounted for 10% of global deaths and in India it probably accounted for over half.

In the mid 20th century, the mortality started dropping, mainly as a result of the spontaneous decline in contact between human and vector populations as a result of improved living conditions as well as by the vector control measures. By the early 1950s, malaria almost disappeared from North America and from almost all of Europe. However, from the tropics where it is endemic, it can spread across continents through the vectors (mosquitoes) and the hosts (men) carried on the boats, trawlers, ships, jets and surface transport.

HISTORY OF MALARIA IN INDIA

Malaria was a serious problem long before India got its independence. Malaria epidemics occurred throughout India with varying intensity. In 1852, one malaria epidemic wiped out the entire village of Ula and then spread across the Bhagirathi river to Hooghly and continued to devastate populations for many years in Burdwan. The development of the Indian railways under the British administration contributed to the spread of malaria. While the construction of railway embankments provided a number of breeding sites for the malaria vectors, the labourers probably introduced different strains of the parasite to the areas in which they worked. Bombay presently called Mumbai suffered greatly from malaria epidemics. The construction of railroads or bridges were often associated with increase in malaria, probably due to imported labour from malarious areas. There were significant outbreaks of malaria during the construction of the Colaba causeway between 1821 and 1841 and during the construction of Alexander Dock and Hughes Dry Dock. Malaria epidemics in Punjab and Bengal both show a startlingly high morbidity and mortality. Bengal suffered a severe malaria epidemic which resulted in over 730,000 deaths in 1921. Thereafter, the number of deaths from malaria slowly decreased to within 300 to 400,000 per annum. However, during the Second World War malaria deaths rose again, particularly in 1943 when Bengal recorded over 680,000 deaths and in 1944 when there were an appalling 763,220 deaths from the disease. Although quinine was available at that time, its supply was probably inadequate and patients did not seek treatment on time.

On the other hand, some of the great successes in controlling the disease were also achieved in India. Formal malaria control programmes were started under British colonial rule and continued after Indian Independence, in 1946. Early malaria control efforts involved removal of breeding sites and later used chemicals such as the larvicides like Paris green and kerosene. One of the first formal operations to control the disease was at Mian Mir, near the city of Lahore (now in Pakistan). Mian Mir had an intricate system of irrigation canals which provided excellent breeding ground for the vectors. The malariologists Dr J.W.W. Stephens and Dr S.R. Christophers, who had worked with Sir Ronald Ross in Freetown, Sierra Leone earlier, arrived at Mian Mir in 1901 with ambitious plans to remove all the breeding sites, evacuate the infected people and administer quinine as both curative and preventative measure. Their programme developed into a massive effort. Between four and five hundred soldiers were set to work full time at filling in the irrigation canals. The programme of constantly filling in ditches and removing puddles and any other potential breeding site continued until 1909. During 1909 there was a serious malaria epidemic, as there was in 1908 throughout the Punjab and the courageous, but ultimately useless control programme was abandoned.

Larviciding operations were also conducted at Bombay, Jhansi, Poona, Meerut, Secunderabad and all other military posts. In 1917, the Bengal Nagpur Railway and the East India Railways formed a separate malaria control organisation, specifically to control the disease in and around stations. National Railways managed to dramatically reduce the incidence of malaria among its staff through a comprehensive larviciding programme. Similar larviciding and breeding pool removal programmes were undertaken during the 1920s in the tea plantations of Assam and in Mysore by the Rockefeller Foundation. In 1927, the Central Malaria Bureau was expanded and renamed as the Malaria Survey of India. The first reported aerial spraying of Paris Green was in 1937. In 1938, pyrethrum was first used in malaria control in Delhi. The Rockefeller Foundation began using pyrethrum sprays experimentally in India to great success. The use of pyrethrum was then expanded to Assam by Dr D. K. Viswanathan in 1942. However, all these interventions were unable to sustain the control of the disease. Vast breeding, colossal number of malaria vectors, limited effectiveness of pyrethrum sprays in houses and cattle sheds against the *An. culicifacies* vector, but not against *An. fluviatilis* and *An. minimus* were some of the causes for this setback.

DDT was first used in India by the armed forces in 1944 for the control of malaria and other vector borne diseases. In 1945, DDT was made available for civilian use in Bombay to control malaria and produced some remarkable results within a very short period. On 1st July 1945, the first civilian home was sprayed in India with a 5% solution of DDT mixed in kerosene. In 1946, pilot schemes using DDT were set up in several areas, including Karnataka, Maharashtra, West Bengal and Assam. Between 1948 and 1952, the WHO set up DDT demonstration teams in Uttar Pradesh, Rayagada, Wynad and Malnad. Use of DDT not only helped in the control of mosquitoes and malaria, but also improved the life expectancy. After the spraying in the Kanara district, the population began to grow because of a decrease in the death rate. Prior to DDT being used, the district reported an average of 50,000 malaria cases every year, which was reduced by around 97% to only 1,500 cases after DDT was introduced. The project was also blessed by Mahatma Gandhi.

During 1949, it was estimated that over 6 million people in Bombay were protected from malaria through the use of DDT and that at least half a million cases of malaria were prevented. In the early 1950s, India's population was estimated to be around 360 million and every year around 75 million people suffered from malaria and approximately 800,000 died from the disease.

Usefulness of DDT prompted the launch of the National Malaria Control Programme (NMCP) in 1953. The control programme first set out to control the disease in the endemic and hyperendemic areas with 125 control units. Each of these control units consisted of between 130 to 275 men and was to protect approximately 1 million people each. By 1958, the malaria control programme had been increased to protect at least 165 million people from the disease with 160 control units. The programme saw tremendous impact and the annual number of cases came down to 49,151 by 1961. With this success, the programme was renamed as National Malaria Eradication Program (NMEP) in 1958 with a belief that malaria could be eradicated in seven to nine years. On the contrary, malaria began to re-emerge in 1965 to reach well over 1 million in 1971. One of the major problems with the eradication programme was that the supervisors could not manage to inspect all of the buildings that had been sprayed. There was a decline in the morale of the spray men and inspectors. With the declining number of cases, complacency set in among spray workers as well as the general population, as people turned the sprayers away. With the incomplete spraying operations, by 1959, resistance to DDT began to develop in certain areas and added to the problem. Furthermore, malaria cases were not treated properly.

With increase in malaria cases in urban areas, The Urban Malaria Scheme (UMS) was launched in 1971 with the objective of controlling malaria by reducing the vector population in the urban areas through recurrent anti-larval measures and detection and treatment of cases through the existing health care services. Passive surveillance (case detection and treatment) and anti-larval measures are the main components of UMS strategy.

The number of malaria cases rose gradually and consistently with a peak of 6.47 million cases in 1976. With this, the focus was again shifted to control of malaria and in 1977, the Modified Plan of Operation (MPO) was launched which also comprised the P. falciparum Containment Programme (PfPC). The objectives of MPO were:

1. Effective control of malaria to reduce malaria morbidity.
2. Prevent deaths due to malaria.
3. Retention of the achievements gained.

Fever Treatment Deport and Drug Distribution Centers were established for distribution of chloroquine. Residual insecticide spray was limited to areas with an API (Annual Parasite Index) above two. By 1985, the incidence rate stabilized at 2 million cases. However, many focal outbreaks, particularly of P. falciparum malaria and deaths from malaria have occurred throughout India since the 1990's and large scale epidemics have been reported from eastern India and Western Rajasthan since 1994. Many of these are related to irrigation projects aided by global funding agencies.

The National Anti Malaria Programme (NAMP) was launched in 1995 as a centrally sponsored scheme on 50:50 cost sharing basis between the centre and the state governments. As the central share, the central government provides drugs, insecticides and larvicides and also technical assistance/guidance as and when required by the state governments. The state governments meet the operational cost including salary of the staff. However, considering the difficulties faced by the seven north-eastern states namely Arunachal Pradesh, Assam, Manipur, Meghalaya, Mizoram, Nagaland and Tripura, 100% central assistance except salary of the staff, which is a non plan activity, is being provided since December, 1994. The union territories without legislatures are also covered under 100% central assistance. An Enhanced Malaria Control Project with World Bank support is being implemented since September, 1997 covering a population of around 62.2

million in 1045 PHCs in 100 predominantly P.falciparum malaria endemic and tribal dominated districts in the peninsular states namely, Andhra Pradesh, Bihar/Jharkhand, Gujarat, Madhya Pradesh/Chattisgarh, Maharashtra, Orissa and Rajasthan. The project lays emphasis on early diagnosis and prompt treatment; selective vector control, eco-friendly methods like introduction of Medicated Mosquito Nets (MMNs), larvivorous fishes, bio-larvicides etc.; epidemic planning and rapid response including inter-sectoral coordination and institutional and human resources development through training/reorientation training; strengthening Management Information System (MIS), Information, Education and Communication (IEC) and operational research. It also aims to cover the most problematic areas and also has the flexibility to divert resources to any needy areas in the country in case of any outbreak of malaria.

In 2004, the integrated National Vector Borne Disease Control Programme (NVBDCP) for the prevention and control of vector borne diseases that is, malaria, dengue, lymphatic filariasis, kala-azar and japanese encephalitis has been launched.

INFORMATIVE NEWSY BRIEFS OF INTEREST

- There are no references to malaria in the 'medical books' of the Mayans or Aztecs. It is likely that European settlers and slavery brought malaria to the New World and the awaiting anophelines within the last 500 years.
- Quinine, a toxic plant alkaloid made from the bark of the Cinchona tree in South America, was used to treat malaria more than 350 years ago
- Jesuit missionaries in South America learned of the anti-malarial properties of the bark of the Cinchona tree and had introduced it into Europe by the 1630s and into India by 1657

- Malaria existed in parts of the United States from colonial times to the 1940s. One of the first military expenditures of the Continental Congress around 1775, was for $300 to buy quinine to protect General Washington's troops.

- In the summer of 1828, 'swamp fever' broke out in the settlement of Bytown (Ottawa) and along the construction route of the Rideau Canal. According to some accounts, the 'malaria' was not native to North America but had been introduced by infected British soldiers who had returned from India. Numerous deaths had occurred by the time the epidemic subsided in September when the mosquitoes disappeared.

- During the American Civil War (1861-1865), one half of the white troops and 80% of the black soldiers of the Union Army got malaria annually

- More than an estimated 600,000 cases of malaria occurred in the U.S. in 1914, according to information from the Center for Disease Control and Prevention in Atlanta, Georgia

- In 1927, J. Wagner von Jauregg was awarded the Nobel Prize in Medicine for his work in treating syphilis using malaria. Patients were inoculated with a type of malaria to produce fevers that would literally burn up the temperature sensitive syphilis bacteria. After three or four cycles of the fever, the patient was administered quinine for a relatively rapid parasitologic cure for the malaria.

- Malaria therapy for syphilis, using monkey and human parasites, continued until the mid1950s when it was replaced by antibiotic chemotherapy

- The Dutch bought cinchona seeds from British trader, Charles Leger, who brought them from Peru. They established cinchona plantations in Java (Indonesia) in the mid 1800s and soon had a virtual monopoly on quinine.

- When the Japanese captured Java during the Second World War, quinine, except for some old stocks became unavailable.

The need for a new synthetic antimalarial became a priority at that time.

- In 1880, a French Army physician, Charles-Louis-Alphonse Laveran, while viewing blood slides under a microscope, made the first true sighting of the malaria parasite in Algeria. The medical community rejected Laveran's discovery and it was not until 1886 that Italian scientists, the leaders in the field at that time, accepted his discovery.
- In 1882, the mosquito transmission hypothesis was first put forward
- The December 18, 1897 issue of the British Medical Journal reported that Dr Ronald Ross discovered malarial cysts in the stomach wall of anopheline mosquitoes that fed on a malaria patient
- By July 1898, malaria transmission through the mosquito was established. At that time, Italian scientist Giovanni Batista Grassi traced the course of the parasite through the mosquito and proved that human malarias were transmitted by species of anopheles.
- Experiments in India in 1932, showed that the monkey malaria, Plasmodium knowlesi, which produced no clinical signs of malaria in Indian rhesus monkeys, was fatal to Malayan irus monkeys and produced a 24 hour fever cycle in humans that terminated in self cure
- Unlike botanical quinine, chloroquine is a synthetically manufactured product that belongs to a class of compounds known as 4-amino quinolines, first developed in 1934 by a German pharmaceutical company
- The first 4-amino quinoline was called Resochin. A slight modification a few years later produced Sontochin. In 1943, the Americans acquired Sontochin when Tunis was liberated

from the Germans. Its composition was again changed slightly and it was renamed Chloroquine.

- 1950 saw the launch of a pilot project for the control of malaria by spraying with DDT

- WHO initiated strategies for the global eradication of malaria in the mid 1950s

- In the 1960s, chloroquine resistant strains of Plasmodium falciparum had arisen; the result of over usage and probably under dosage. At that time, there was no drug to treat chloroquine resistant malaria except the ancient antimalarial, quinine.

- By 1966, it had been shown that 10 species of Plasmodium, naturally present in monkeys and apes, were capable of infecting humans. Often an infection in one species that produces no clinical signs of malaria can cause severe illness and death when transferred, through inoculation, to another.

- Quinine has now been completely synthesised. Its synthetic analogue is called mefloquine.

- A 'new' antimalarial drug is called Qinghaosu, which is derived from the sweet wonnwood (Qinghao) plant (genus Artemisia). It has been used in China for more than two thousand years to treat fever associated with malaria. The drug has been shown to be effective in the treatment of the most deadly forms of falciparum malaria and has been effective against strains of Plasmodium falciparum that are solidly resistant to chloroquine.

- From 1956 to 1969, the United States, through the U.S. Agency for International Aid, (USAID) gave $790 million to the Global Eradication of Malaria Programme. From 1955 to about 1970, USAID gave approximately $1 billion to WHO and various National Malaria Eradication Programmes.

- In 1967, WHO realised that the global eradication of malaria was impossible for a variety of reasons and the focus shifted to control of the deadly disease. In 1972, the Global Eradication of Malaria Programme was formally declared dead.
- In 1987, Dr Manuel Elkin Patarroyo, a biochemist from Colombia, developed the first synthetic vaccine against the Plasmodium falciparum parasite. The vaccine is still being developed and has not yet proven to reduce deaths in Africa. In 1992, Dr Patarroyo donated the vaccine to the World Health Organisation.

Malaria – Marred

- Alexander the Great, in alliance with Greek states, had conquered the Persians, capturing the entire coastline of the eastern Mediterranean, Syria, Phoenicia, Arabia, Egypt and valiant tribes of northern India, virtually conquering the entire known world. When he was about to depart with his army in early June 323 B.C. to subjugate the earth, he contracted a fever and the voyage was postponed. At first the 33 years old general regarded his illness as nothing more than a temporary setback. But Alexander continued to deteriorate until he lapsed into a deep coma and died. Malaria, by striking Alexander, had altered the course of history.
- In the fourth century A.D., Alaric, King of the Goths, attacked Rome and triumphed. But his triumph was short lived for he got sick with malaria and died soon after entering the town.
- The invading army of Attila (452 A.D.) was stopped in Rome by malaria
- Emperor Otto I attacked Rome in 964 to suppress a revolt there but almost all his men died of malaria. On 7 Dec., 983, his eldest son, Otto II, died of malaria at the age of 28 years in spite of medical intervention.

- Frederick I, called Barbarossa, also failed in his attempt to conquer Rome. The army of Henry II was wiped out by malaria, but Henry IV managed to besiege Rome four times, always withdrawing the bulk of his soldiers during the summer months from the Campagna. The tiny force left behind was invariably annihilated by fever.

- Malaria probably played a part in dissuading Genghis Khan (1162-1227) from invading Western Europe

- After the death of Pope Alexander VI in 1503, his son Cesare Borgia plotted to dominate all Italy. But shortly, Cesare contracted severe malaria and was saved by his family doctor. By the time Cesare Borgia recoverd, his opportunity had passed.

- By the end of 15th century, Columbus dropped anchor at the site of an old Indian village on Hispaniola to build a fort and colony on his second voyage to the New World. After a month, an epidemic of terrible fever afflicted the entire party, including Columbus himself.

- One of the first military expenditures of the Continental Congress, around 1775, was for $300 to buy quinine to protect General Washington's troops

- Malaria and yellow fever kept Napoleon Bonaparte from putting down the uprising in Hati in 1801

- July 30, 1809 a British armed force of 39,000 men landed on Walcheren with a view to assisting the Austrians in their war against Napoleon and attacking the French fleet moored at Flushing (Vlissingen). Napoleon had consolidated his grip on the continent by defeating the Austrians at Wagram earlier in the month. Napoleon reportedly flooded the Holland countryside to allow malaria to become rampant. Napoleon reportedly stated: 'We must oppose the English with nothing but fever, which will soon devour them all.' During the

American civil war in 1861-1865, malaria accounted for 1,316,000 episodes of illness and 10,000 deaths. It has been estimated that 50% of the white soldiers and 80% of the black soldiers got malaria annually.

- The French campaign in Madagascar in 1895 saw 13 deaths in action and over 4,000 deaths due to malaria
- **World War I**: In Macedonia, British, French and German armies were immobilised for 3 years by malaria. On one occasion, when the French commanding general was ordered to attack, he replied, 'Regret that my army is in hospital with malaria.' Nearly 80 percent of 120,000 French troops in this area were hospitalised with malaria. Approximately 7.5/1,000 Americans quartered in the U.S. were infected with malaria in 1917.
- **World War II**: Many troops had to suffer casualties by inflicted malaria. Gen. Douglas MacArthur's predicament in May 1943 is very clear: 'This will be a long war if for every division I have facing the enemy I must count on a second division in hospital with malaria and a third division convalescing from this debilitating disease!' It appears that the general was not at all worried about defeating the Japanese, but was greatly concerned about the failure to defeat the anopheles mosquito. 60,000 U.S. troops died in Africa and the South Pacific from malaria.
- Development and use of synthetic antimalarial drugs and residual insecticides like DDT were greatest contributions to malariology from World War II. The dependency on quinine as the only antimalarial was relieved and many new antimalarials like chloroquine, amodiaquine, primaquine, proquanil and pyrimethamine came into use.
- **Korean War (1950-1953)**: U.S. military hospitals were full with cases of malaria, with as many as 629 cases per week.

More than 3,000 cases of malaria were documented in U.S. troops that served during the war.

- **Vietnam War (1962–1975)**: Malaria victimised more combatants during the war than bullets. The disease reduced the combat strength of some units by half. The U.S. Army established a malaria drug research program when U.S. troops first encountered drug resistant malaria during the war. In 1967, the Chinese scientists set up Project 523, a secret military project to help the Vietnamese military defeat malaria by developing artemisinin based anti malarial formulations.

- **Operation Restore Hope (1992–1994)**: Malaria was the No. 1 cause of casualties among U.S. troops during the operation. From the time of deployment through April 1993, malaria was diagnosed in 48 military personnel. Malaria was diagnosed in 83 military personnel (21 Marine and 62 Army) following their return from Somalia.

- **Malaria in Afghanistan, Iraq and Liberia (2001–2003)**: Many US soldiers in Iraq walked while eating just to avoid being bitten and infected by mosquitoes. In October 2001, a falciparum malaria epidemic that erupted in Afghanistan claimed 53 lives. When 290 marines went ashore in Liberia in September 2003, 80 contracted malaria. Of the 157 troops who spent at least one night ashore, 69 became infected. In Liberia, over a third of U.S. marines sent in as military advisors to oversee a civil transition have contracted malaria.

- Malaria has posed major problems during natural calamities. Outbreaks of malaria was a problem during many major constructions like that of the Suez canal and the Panama Canal. The Vatican was moved from a lower lying area to its present location, with work beginning in 1574, due to malaria. Malaria continues to be a challenge in such situations even today.

EPIDEMIOLOGY

MALARIA is the second most deadly infection in the world, next to tuberculosis. In the world, maximum number of patients are in Africa. In India it is seen in regions of Orissa, Jharkhand, Chhattisgarh, Assam, Madhya Pradesh, Rajasthan and the largest number of deaths are reported in Assam, Orissa, West Bengal, Arunachal Pradesh, Meghalaya, Maharashtra, Mizoram, Gujarat, and Karnataka. This infection is present throughout the world, like in Asia, parts of Greece, Turkey, Middle East, Central and South America. People who live in an endemic area acquire a degree of immunity, which decreases with time. High risk groups are travellers, emigrants returning home from a long spell abroad whose immunity has elapsed, pregnant women, and immunosuppressed patients.

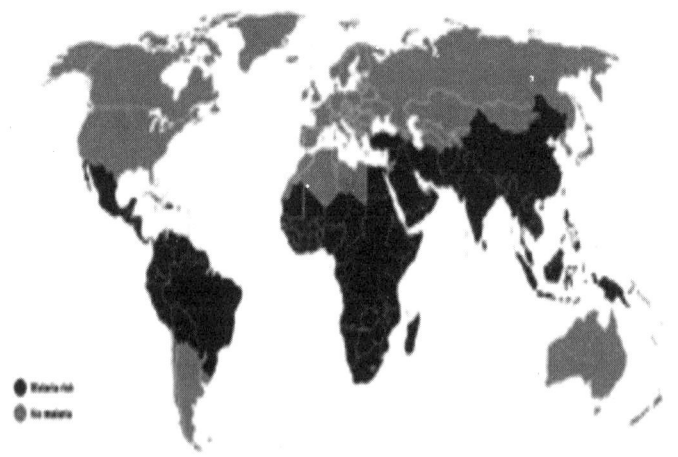

Dark area – malaria endemic areas

History and Epidemiology ■ 55

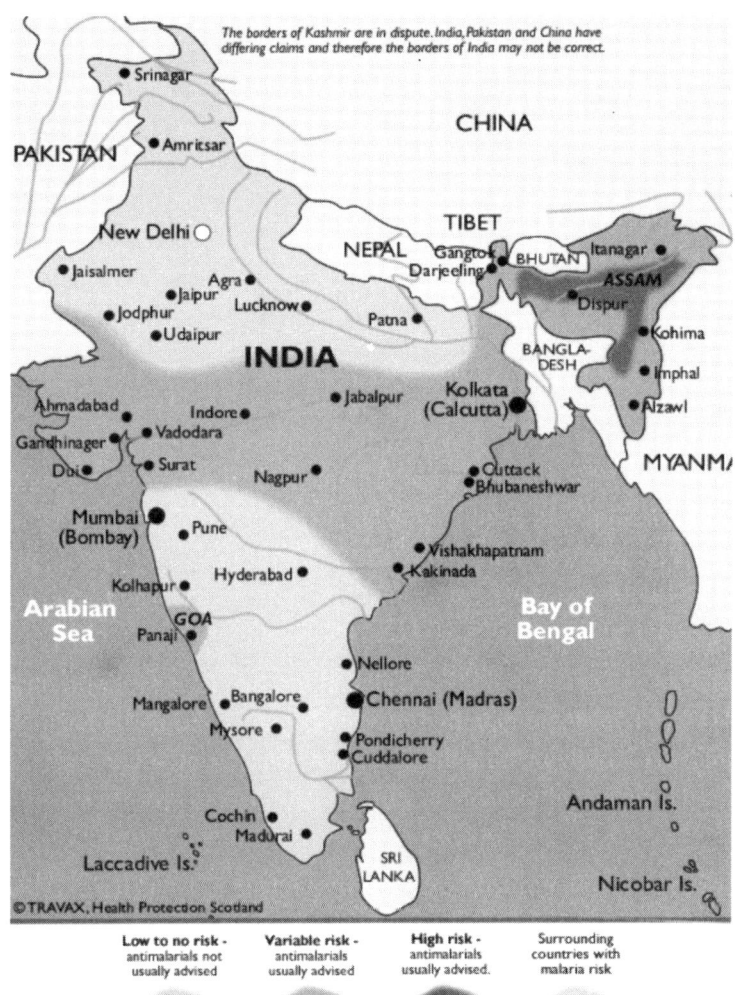

This map is only intended as a guide since mosquitoes do not respect boundaries and the risk areas shown may not be exact.

Chapter 5

Clinical Presentation

ETIOLOGY

Malaria is caused by infection with a parasite called Plasmodium that is transmitted by mosquitoes. In the human body, the parasites multiply in the liver, and then infect red blood cells. Usually, people get malaria by being bitten by an infective female anopheles mosquito. Only anopheles mosquitoes can transmit malaria and they must have been infected through a previous blood meal taken on an infected person. When a mosquito bites an infected person, a small amount of blood is taken which contains microscopic malaria parasites. About 1 week later, when the mosquito takes its next blood meal, these parasites mix with the mosquito's saliva and are injected into the person being bitten. Because the malaria parasite is found in red blood cells of an infected person, malaria can also be transmitted through blood transfusion, organ transplant, or the shared use of needles or syringes contaminated with blood. Malaria may also be transmitted from a mother to her unborn infant before or during delivery then it is called congenital malaria.

Source of Infection

Patient, parasite carrier

Route of Transmission

- Female mosquito biting person
- Blood transfusion

Susceptibility

- Universal susceptibility
- No cross immunity
- Re-infection

Epidemic Features

Sporadic or endemic, tropic or subtropics

Causative organism

- P. vivax: Tertian malaria
- P. malariae: Quartan malaria
- P. falciparum: Malignant malaria
- P. ovale: Tertian malaria

Etiology

The malaria is caused by:

- Tachysporozoite
- Bradysporozoite
- Merozoites
- Sporozoites
- Parasitemia

PATHOGENESIS

The pathology of malaria fever depends upon the type of parasite causing the infection.

Pathogenicity: merozoites, malarial pigment and products of metabolism.

Two phases:

Human - whole asexual reproduction

Mosquito - sexual parasitic stage

Two hosts:

Human - intermediate host

Mosquito - final host

The presentation of the symptomatology is according to the stage of the mosquito life cycle:

The clinical symptoms are seen in the erythrocytic stage.

The relapse of the fever occurs in the exo-erythrocytic stage.

The infectivity is seen in the sporozoites.

Pathologically malaria fever is of two types—Benign and Malignant.

Benign malaria is caused due to the infection of the Plasmodium ovale, Plasmodium vivax and the Plasmodium malariae.

Malignant malaria is caused by the Plasmodium falciparum.

Mechanism of attack by the plasmodium is as follows:

1. RBC rupture affects the merozoites, which release the malaria pigment. The products of metabolism enter the blood circulation and produce the allergy like symptoms.
2. P. falciparum affects the end arteries hence produces micro vascular diseases and the magnitude of parasitemia is directly proportionate to the age / health status of the patient, with no specific antibodies or cell mediated response.

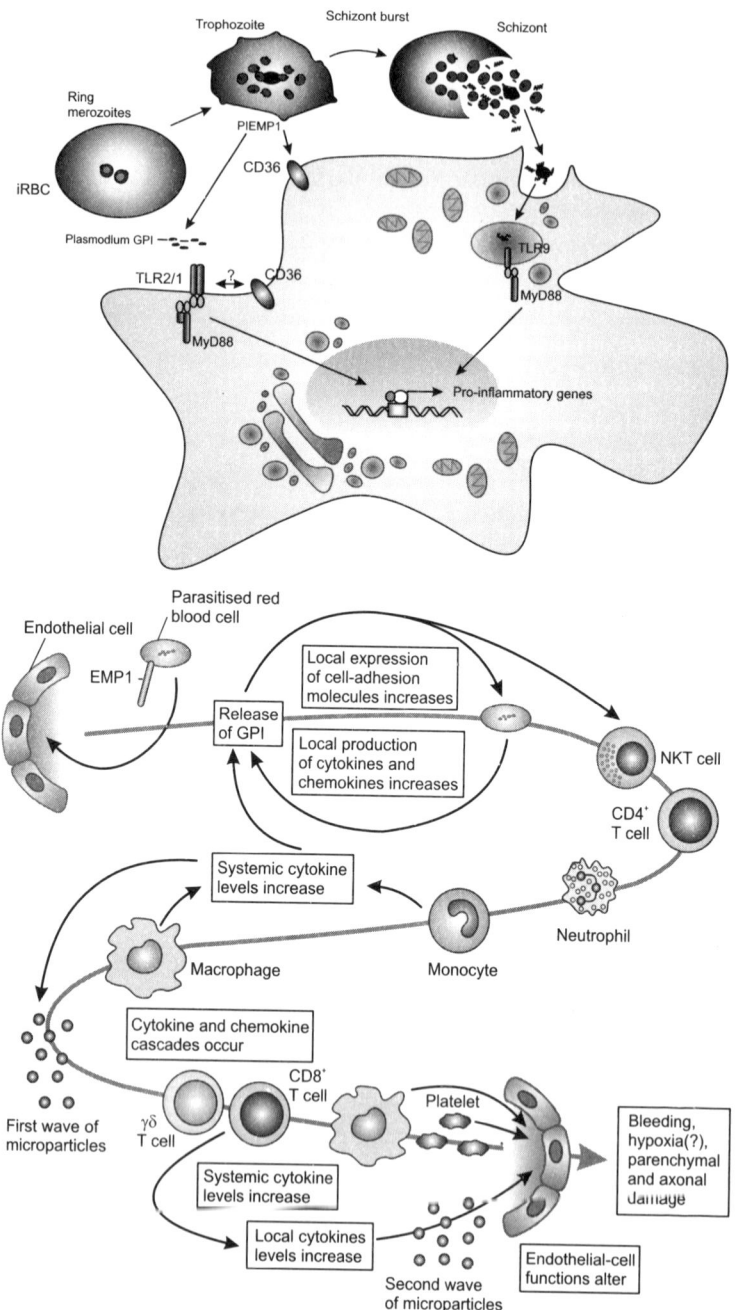

First, parasitised red blood cells (PRBCs) adhere to receptors expressed by brain micro vascular endothelial cells, such as intercellular adhesion molecule 1 (ICAM1), through surface expression of Plasmodium falciparum erythrocyte membrane protein 1 (EMP1). When merozoites are released from PRBCs 4 hours later, parasite glycosylphosphatidylinositol (GPI), which is either released into the blood or present in parasite membranes, functions as a pathogen-associated molecular pattern and toxin, thereby inducing an inflammatory response. A local acute-phase response then occurs, which involves activation of the endothelium and local production of cytokines and chemokines, and this result in up regulation of expression of cell adhesion molecules by endothelial cells. Within the next 24 hours, this cycle is perpetuated and exacerbated, owing to increasing parasite numbers and further binding of PRBCs to endothelial cells that have upregulated expression of cell adhesion molecules. GPI can also function as a ligand for CD1d-restricted natural killer T (NKT) cells, leading to their activation. Activated NKT cells can regulate the differentiation of CD4+ T cells into T helper 1 (TH1) or TH2 cells, depending on which natural killer complex loci are expressed, so activation and involvement of CD4+ T cells occurs. In addition, chemokines recruit monocytes and activate neutrophils (although neutrophils are not known to infiltrate brain microvessels in humans or mice with cerebral malaria). Recruited monocytes can then differentiate into macrophages and become arrested in brain microvessels. Macrophages can also be activated by GPI, a process that is amplified by interferon. Local activated macrophages produce more chemokines, which are released systemically, thereby amplifying infiltration of cells, sequestration of PRBCs and release of microparticles (which are probably of endothelial cell origin). After several more cycles, T cells and CD8+ T cells might become involved, releasing more chemokines and cytokines both systemically and locally and possibly inducing perforin mediated lesions in the endothelium. Together with locally arrested macrophages, platelets are sequestered and participate in altering endothelial cell functions. More microparticles of platelet, endothelial cell and monocyte origin are released, which leads to the dissemination of pro-inflammatory and pro-coagulant effects. Finally, damage to the endothelium, with possible perivascular haemorrhage, axonal injury, and neurotransmitter and metabolic changes, can ensue. The overall disease spectrum in humans might depend on whether all of these processes occur or only some of them.

When the infection is caused then the pathogenesis is seen in the following organs / systems.

1. Gastro intestinal tract
2. Spleen
3. Liver
4. Genitourinary system
5. Respiratory system
6. Cardiovascular system
7. Brain
8. Blood

Result of complex interactions within vasculature mediated by humoral, vascular and hematological factors. An immune mediated inflammatory reaction releases vasoactive products, which cause endothelial damage.

Trophozoites within RBCs induce changes in RBCs as trophozoites mature that makes them capable of adhering to vascular endothelium. This results in sequestration of RBCs in small cerebral venules, micro vascular congestion and tissue hypoxia. It is not clear whether cerebral oedema plays a significant role.

Hypoglycemia is an important complication of cerebral malaria and may contribute to decreased level of consciousness.

Gastrointestinal Tract

It is composed of mouth, oesophagus, stomach, intestines, rectum and anal canal.

In a patient suffering from malaria the taste becomes bitter, and nausea and vomiting is a common feature. There is pain in the epigastrium, distension of the abdomen and this may be associated with loose stools.

The symptoms due to P.ovale, P.vivax and P. malariae are usually of mild character, whereas in cases of P. falciparum there is necrosis and blockage of the intestinal arteries which causes ischaemia, ulceration and oedema. These symptoms may lead to sepsis if there is delay in diagnosing the malaria parasite.

Spleen

The spleen is located in the upper left part of the abdomen, the largest of the body's ductless glands. It is an oval flattened organ and normally has a dull purple color. It has a convex or parietal surface which lies against the diaphragmatic concavity and a concave visceral surface.

The most important function of the spleen is to produce lymphocytes for strengthening the immune system. The other function is to remove all the old red blood cells from the circulation, storage and production of white blood cells.

The enlargement of spleen occurs in the first attack of fever due to the enlargement of the blood vessels, edema and hyperplasia of the tissues. This causes increased hemolytic and phagocytic activity of the spleen.

If the treatment is provided in proper dose and time then the spleen returns to its normal size in 2 weeks. Or it becomes non palpable.

Except the P.falciparum all varieties of the Plasmodium cause enlargement of the spleen in first paroxysm of fever.

In cases of repeated malarial fevers, the spleen returns to its normal size slowly due to the chronicity of the disease process.

Normal weight of spleen is 150 gms and length is 11 cm.

An example of the disease affecting spleen which is caused due to malaria is tropical splenomegaly syndrome. In this, the weight of the spleen increases up to 2000 to 44,000 gms (normal weight-150 gms), there occurs enlargement of the spleen, increased phagocytosis of red blood cells and white blood cells. The levels of IgG, IgM antibodies against malaria are present.

Liver

The enlargement of the liver occurs along with that of the spleen. On palpation the liver is firm and tender. Whereas if seen under microscope it is brown or black in colour due to the deposition of the malarial parasites.

Histologically, sinusoides are dilated with hypertrophied kupffer cells and parasitised red cells around them. Central part of the lobes show necrosis.

In P.malariae the symptoms are similar to that of nephritic syndrome characterised by albuminuria, swelling of the upper eyelids and face, and hypertension.

In P.falciparum the symptoms arise due to the occlusion of the end arteries of the kidney causing necrosis of the glomeruli and the renal tubules.

Genitourinary System

The main organs of this system are kidneys, ureters and urinary bladder.

The kidneys are the main organs for the excretion of the urine.

In P.malariae the symptoms are similar to that of nephritic syndrome characterised by albuminuria, swelling of the upper eyelids and face, and hypertension.

In P.falciparum the symptoms arise due to the occlusion of the end arteries of the kidney causing necrosis of the glomeruli and the renal tubules.

Respiratory System

The organs of respiratory system are the trachea and the lungs.

In P.falciparum due to the occlusion of the micro arteries there are seen endothelial lesions and perivascular edema. This results in pulmonary edema and the sputum is of pink colour. There is respiratory distress which further complicates the condition of the patient.

Cardiovascular System

The heart and the major vessels constitute the cardiovascular system.

The P. falciparum causes changes in the coronary arteries and the myocardial vessels become congested due to the deposition of the parasitised red cells, macrophages having malarial pigments, lymphocytes and plasma cells. This results in obstruction of the valve and cardiac failure due to impairment of the circulation.

Signs and symptoms include fast pulse with miffed heart sounds, transient systolic murmur at the apex due to cardiac dilatation, cyanosis of the extremities, hands and feet are cold to touch and blood pressure is low.

White blood cells recognize the plasmodium infected erythrocytes and phagocytose them. This leads to their accumulation into the spleen which becomes enlarged and turns black because of the high load of undigestible malaria pigment.

Brain

The P.falciparum causes occlusion of the arteries of the brain resulting in lack of oxygen to the brain. The granulomas and hemorrhages in the brain produce malarial encephalitis and meningoencephalitis.

The symptoms are headache, vomiting, delirium and anxiety along with the paroxysm of the fever.

Blood

The type of red blood cell which is affected in the malarial patient by the species is:

P. vivax infects the retiform red blood cell.

P. malariae infects the mature red blood cell.

P. falciparum infects each and every red blood cell.

SIGNS AND SYMPTOMS

The symptoms begin 10 days to 4 weeks after infection, although it can be seen as early as 7 days or as late as 1 year.

Two kinds of malaria caused by P. vivax and P. ovale can occur again (relapsing malaria).

In P. vivax and P. ovale infections, some parasites can remain dormant in the liver for several months up to about 4 years after a person is bitten by an infected mosquito. When these parasites come out of hibernation and begin invading red blood cells the person will become sick again.

Infection with malarial parasites may result in a wide variety of symptoms, ranging from absent or very mild symptoms to severe disease and even death.

Malaria disease can be categorized as uncomplicated or complicated.

There are three types of malarial fever that may be classified as:

1. Tertian Fever
2. Quartan Fever
3. Malignant Fever

Tertian Fever: The attacks surface on alternate days. Caused by P. falciparum, P. vivax, and P. ovale.

Quartan Fever: In this fever the attack of fever occurs after an interval of two days, i.e. if first attack of fever occurs on the first, another attack will occur on the 4th day, then 7th, 9th and so on. Caused by P. malariae.

Malignant Fever: It is a variety of severe type of malarial fever when malignancy sets in and is, thus, the most severe and most alarming type of malarial fever.

Incubation period

Quartan malaria: 24-30 days

Tertian malaria: 13-15 days

Malignant malaria: 7-12 days

Mild early symptoms appear in few days before major symptoms like:

Headache, pain in muscles, pain in abdomen, weakness and lethargy or tired feeling in the whole body.

This may last for 1-2 days after that comes the typical chills stage, fever stage and lastly the marked perspiration, which leads to fall in temperature.

Cold stage: Fever up to 40°C, shaking chills.

Hot stage: High fever, headache, nausea, vomiting, dizziness, pain in whole body and delirium.

Sweating stage: Sweating followed by fall in temperature and prostration.

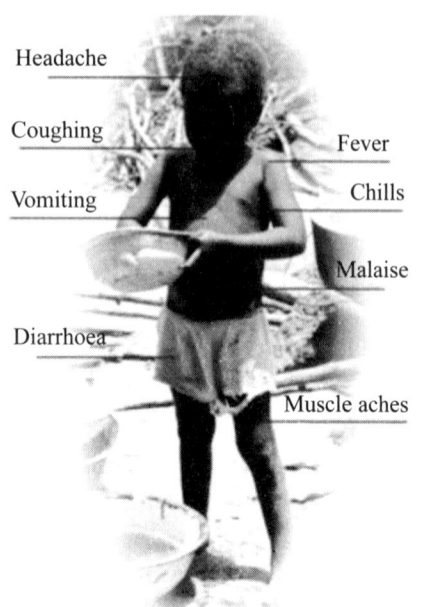

Signs

- Anaemia
- Pallor
- Tiredness
- Fatigue
- Shortness of breath
- Splenomegaly
- Hepatomegaly
- Elevated ALT- serum Alanine aminotransferase

Plasmodium vivax: Stays in the liver for up to three years and can lead to a relapse.

Plasmodium ovale: Stays in blood and liver for many years without causing symptoms.

Plasmodium falciparum: This is the only parasite that causes malignant malaria.

Plasmodium malariae: This causes benign malaria and is relatively rare.

Symptoms

Cold Stage

As the temperature begins to rise, there is intense headache and muscular discomfort. The patient feels cold, wants many blankets, and curls up shivering. The shaking of the body due to chills last for 10-30 minutes but can last up to 90 minutes, followed by a rise in body temperature.

Hot Stage

By the end of the cold stage the extremities become hot and skin becomes dry.

Sweating

Profuse sweat then breaks out. It lasts for 2-4 hours. The patient is soaked in sweat and the temp falls. Blood pressure is relatively low. The patient feels exhausted and may sleep. Defervescence usually takes 4-8 hours. Fever is irregular at first with temperature exceeding 39 degrees centigrade. It may rise up to 40°C.

If a mosquito carrying the P. falciparum parasite bites one, then the symptoms usually appear within three months of being bitten.

If a mosquito carrying the P. vivax, P. ovale or P. malariae parasite, then the symptoms can appear a year or more after being bitten, because the parasite can lay dormant in the liver and become active months later. More commonly, the patient presents with a combination of the following symptoms:

- Fever
- Chill
- Sweat
- Headache
- Nausea and vomiting
- Body ache
- General malaise

In countries where cases of malaria are infrequent, these symptoms may be attributed to influenza, a cold, or other common infections, especially if malaria is not suspected. Conversely, in countries where malaria is frequent, residents often recognize the symptoms as malaria and treat themselves without seeking diagnostic confirmation.

Physical findings are:

1. Elevated temperature
2. Perspiration
3. Weakness
4. Enlarged spleen

In P. falciparum malaria, additional findings are:

1. Mild jaundice
2. Enlargement of the liver
3. Increased respiratory rate

Diagnosis of malaria depends on the demonstration of parasites on a blood smear examined under a microscope.

In P. falciparum malaria, additional laboratory findings are:

i. Mild anaemia

ii. Mild decrease in blood platelets or thrombocytopenia

iii. Elevation of bilirubin

iv. Elevation of aminotransferase

v. Albuminuria

vi. Presence of abnormal bodies in the urine

Severe Malaria

Severe malaria occurs when P. falciparum infections are complicated by serious organ failures or abnormalities in the patient's blood or metabolism. The manifestations of severe malaria are:

Cerebral malaria

Patient presents with abnormal behaviour, impairment of consciousness, seizures, coma or other neurological abnormalities.

Severe anemia due to hemolysis (destruction of the red blood cells).

Hemoglobinuria (hemoglobin in the urine) due to hemolysis

Pulmonary oedema (fluid buildup in the lungs) or acute respiratory distress syndrome (ARDS), which may occur even after the parasite counts have decreased in response to treatment. Abnormalities in blood coagulation and thrombocytopenia (decrease in blood platelets), cardiovascular collapse and shock.

Acute Kidney Failure

Hyperparasitemia, where more than 5% of the red blood cells are infected by malarial parasites.

Metabolic acidosis, a condition where there is excessive acidity in the blood and tissue fluids.

Hypoglycaemia is a condition of low blood glucose. Hypoglycaemia may also occur in pregnant women with uncomplicated malaria, or after treatment with quinine.

Severe malaria occurs most often in persons who have no immunity to malaria or whose immunity has decreased.

These include all residents of areas with low or no malaria transmission, and young children and pregnant women in areas with high transmission. In all areas, severe malaria is a medical emergency and should be treated urgently and aggressively.

Malaria Relapses

In P. vivax and P. ovale infections, patients having recovered from the first episode of illness may suffer several additional attacks after months or even years without symptoms, because P. vivax and P. ovale have dormant liver stage parasites, hypnozoites that may reactivate. Neurological defects may occasionally persist following cerebral malaria, especially in children, like ataxia, palsies, speech difficulties, deafness, and blindness. P. vivax malaria can cause rupture of the spleen or acute respiratory distress syndrome.

Recurrent infections with P. falciparum may result in severe anaemia.

Malaria during pregnancy especially P. falciparum may cause severe disease in the mother, and may lead to premature delivery or delivery of a low birth weight baby.

Nephrotic syndrome, a chronic, severe kidney disease can result from chronic or repeated infections with P. malariae.

When malaria is caused by blood transfusion its incubation period is 7-10 days. There are no exoerythrogenic phase and no relapses of the disease.

COMPLICATIONS

Malaria can potentially be a very serious illness and in some cases, it can be fatal. The falciparum strain of the plasmodium parasite causes the most severe malarial symptoms and results in the most fatalities.

Anaemia

The extensive destruction of red blood cells can cause severe anaemia.

Cerebral Malaria

The infected red blood cells block the small blood vessels leading to the brain causing necrosis, swelling of the brain and this leads to permanent brain damage, seizures and coma.

Systemic Complications

- Breathing problems
- Dehydration
- Liver failure
- Shock
- Spontaneous bleeding
- Jaundice
- Hypoglycemia
- Kidney failure
- Swelling and rupturing of the spleen

Complications of malaria tend to be more severe in pregnant women and children.

The complications of benign malaria are of mild character and affect spleen, liver, blood and kidneys.

The complications of malignant malaria due to P.falciparum occur gradually after many days of fever and affects brain and other organs in a fatal way.

There are certain factors which are present in the patient when he is infected by the P.falciparum which will complicate the malarial fever, such as:

1. Age of the patient.
2. Pregnancy-second trimester of pregnancy.
3. Pre-existing diseases for which the patient is taking steroids, anti-cancer and anti-tuberculosis treatments.
4. Patients who have undergone removal of spleen.
5. Lack of previous malarial infections.

Defining Features of Severe Malaria as Published by the World Health Organization

1. Coma (Blantyre Coma Scale 2)*
2. Seizure (one or more witnessed by the investigators)
3. Obtundation (depressed consciousness with BCS > 2)
4. Parasitemia 500,000/mm3
5. Lethargy or prostration (clinical judgment or child 7 months old unable to sit unassisted)
6. Severe anaemia (hemoglobin 5 g/dL)
7. Respiratory distress (intercostal muscle retraction, deep breathing, grunting)
8. Hypoglycaemia (glucose 40 mg/dL)

9. Jaundice
10. Renal insufficiency as indicated by lack of urination for 1 day
11. Gross hematuria
12. Inability to eat or drink
13. State of shock (systolic blood pressure 50 mm of Hg, rapid pulse, cold extremities)
14. Repeated vomiting

[* The scale uses motor and crying responses to pain and includes the ability to watch. It can be used to assess young children with cerebral malaria.]

Response	Findings	Score
Best motor response	localizes painful stimulus (pressure with blunt end of pencil on sternum or supraorbital ridge)	2
	withdraws limb from painful stimulus (pressure with horizontal pencil on nail bed of finger or toe)	1
	no response or inappropriate response	0
Best verbal response	cries appropriately with painful stimulus, or, if verbal, speaks	2
	moan or abnormal cry with painful stimulus	1
	no vocal response to painful stimulus	0
Eye movement	watches or follows (e.g., mother's face)	1
	fails to watch or follow	0

Blantyre coma scale = (Best motor response score) + (best verbal response score) + (eye movement score)

Interpretation:
- Minimum score: 0 (poor)
- Maximum score: 5 (good)
- Abnormal score: <= 4

DIFFERENTIAL DIAGNOSIS

Misdiagnosis

The disease process is either by over treatment or under treatment tends to delay the relief and cure, this may lead to complications.

Under Treatment

There are certain conditions when the treatment gets delayed due to the following factors:

1. Delay in starting treatment, waiting for the proper diagnosis.
2. Withholding antimalarial drug for fear of toxicity.
3. Inadequate dosage. If a proper dosage is not given then the malaria will not be checked.
4. Miscalculation of the dose due to base-salt confusion.
5. Failure to identify the need for parenteral therapy in severe malaria and to identify. Therapeutic priorities in severe malaria.
6. Oral therapy in severe malaria.
7. Stopping antimalarial therapy for minor side effects is unjustified. Always weigh the benefits and risks.
8. Failure to control convulsions.

9. Failure to recognize and treat severe anaemia.
10. Delay in starting mechanical ventilation in patients with ARDS, metabolic acidosis etc.
11. Delay in starting dialysis in cases of renal failure.
12. Delay in considering obstetrical intervention.

Over Treatment

1. Use of parenteral antimalarial when not needed it can cause unnecessary hardship to patient.
2. Using 2nd line antimalarial when not indicated. This only adds to the cost of therapy and to the adverse effects. It also depletes our stock of reserve antimalarial drugs and exposes them to the risk of development of resistance.
3. Using 2-3 antimalarial drugs concurrently.
4. Higher dose and longer duration: Antimalarial drugs do not offer better efficacy at higher dose, this only adds to the adverse effects.
5. Failure to switch to oral therapy: Unnecessary continuation of parenteral therapy may increase the adverse effects and also cost of therapy.
6. Rapid intravenous infusions of Chloroquine and quinine may be fatal.
7. Over hydration and fluid overload: Enthusiastic administration of fluid and/or blood may precipitate acute pulmonary oedema.
8. Unnecessary endotracheal intubation in comatose patients who can be managed with conservative measures.

PROGNOSIS

The outcome is expected to be good in most cases of malaria with treatment, but poor in falciparum infection with complications.

Malaria can kill within 24 hours, if the treatment is not started immediately.

Mortality rate is 25-50% with treatment. Delay in treatment is major factor contributing to poor outcome.

Clinical features which suggest poor prognosis

1. Impaired consciousness. The deeper the coma the worse the prognosis.
2. 3 or more convulsions within 24 hours
3. Respiratory distress
4. Substantial bleeding
5. Shock

The Laboratory findings which show a Poor Prognosis of the Disease

Blood Test

1. Creatinine 265 mmol/l or more
2. Bilirubin >43 mmol/l. Combination of deep jaundice and renal failure associated with a particularly grave prognosis.
3. Metabolic acidosis (bicarbonate <15 mmol/l)
4. Hyperlactatemia (venous lacate >5 mmol/l)
5. Hypoglycaemia
6. Aminotransferase >3 times normal

7. Parasitemia (>500,000 parasites/ml or >10,000 mature trophozoites and schizonts/ml) Trophozoites are mature parasites in which pigment is visible under light microscopy. 5% of neutrophils contain malaria parasite.

Chapter 6

Malaria Associated with Other Diseases

MALARIA IN PREGNANCY

Malaria can affect in all the trimesters of pregnancy because the immune system is weak during the pregnancy and the body is less able to fight off the bacteria and the infections. The effects of malaria on the foetus can be from simple miscarriage to still birth, premature delivery, low birth weight and death of the foetus. Complications are more in the first and second pregnancies. Later on, the immunity develops and the effects are less serious then.

The drug which can be prescribed during pregnancy, should be as per national drug policy.

Signs and Symptoms

The presentations are atypical in second and third trimesters.

Fever can have different patterns like low grade, high grade or no fever at all.

A travel history should always be taken in pregnant woman who presents with fever and anemia.

Splenomegaly is present but it regresses in later half of the pregnancy.

Anaemia is present and becomes more severe with pregnancy.

Cerebral malaria is presented as seizures, impaired consciousness and coma.

Complications

In the mother:

1. Anaemia occurs between 16-29 weeks. This is due to destruction of parasitised cells and increased demands of pregnancy.
2. Acute pulmonary oedema occurs in second and third trimesters. It is considered as a high mortality for the mother.
3. Hypoglycaemia: This is much more common in pregnancy. It can be aggravated by treatment with parenteral quinine.
4. Cerebral malaria is much common in pregnant women.
5. Disseminated intravascular coagulation can occur and carries a high mortality.
6. In endemic/high transmission areas for malaria, baseline immunity to malaria is decreased by pregnancy.

In the foetus:

1. Spontaneous abortion
2. Low birth weight
3. Intra uterine growth retardation
4. Still births
5. Premature delivery

In the infants:

1. Congenital malaria

2. Anaemia
3. More prone to other infections
4. Under nutrition
5. Increased mortality rates

Congenital Malaria

This occurs due to the transplacental spread from non immune mothers who have malaria during pregnancy. The symptoms are fever, feeding difficulties, jaundice, anaemia, hepatosplenomegaly and mental irritability in the infants.

The most important thing is one should always consider a congenital malaria in an infant with fever in first three months of life, whose mother has traveled to or migrated from malarial regions.

Placental Malaria

Placental malaria occurs when the red blood cells are infected by Plasmodium falciparum and get accumulated in the intervillous space of the placenta.

Treatment

Treatment should be given according to the clinical conditions, local resistance pattern of the patient where she is residing, and the dosage. The most important is the usage of a safe drug during pregnancy.

Following drugs can be used in pregnancy:

1. Chloroquine and Quinine are safe in all the trimesters, but the resistance is common.
2. Artimesinins can be safe in the second and third trimesters.

3. Mefloquine and pyrimethamine/sulphadoxine are safe in second and third trimesters.
4. Primaquine, tetracycline, doxycycline and halofantrine are contraindicated.

MALARIA IN HIV/AIDS

Both diseases kill millions of people each year, and both diseases are scourges of developing nations in Africa, South Asia, Southeast Asia and South America. But HIV is pandemic, spread from person to person by sexual contact in an increasingly mobile world. Malaria is endemic, dependent on a local symbiosis between infected female anophele mosquitoes and humans. The severe symptoms of malaria caused by the tiny parasite Plasmodium falciparum appear within days and bring death to about 15 to 25% of those stricken when great quantities of infected red blood cells are destroyed in a single burst. HIV infection is a slow, insidious process that can take years to deplete immunologically crucial white blood cells. AIDS results in death for nearly all untreated patients.

Both diseases can be transmitted by contaminated blood. In the eighties, some partially blamed the initial spread of HIV in Africa on the transfusion of infected blood to treat malaria associated anemia. And a study in Brazil has tracked an outbreak of blood-borne malaria among urban HIV infected intravenous drug users. (Bastos)

The infection rate of both diseases can be reduced by behavior changes, barrier protection (condoms or bed nets) and medical prophylaxis. Vaccine development for both diseases has been slow. But malaria can often be treated and cured with an inexpensive weeklong course of drugs whereas current HIV treatment is a lifelong prospect of daily medication at costs that have so far limited their use in developing countries. Most people who contract HIV or malaria are poor.

With shared geography and demographics, co-infection is common, yet surprisingly few obvious clinical associations between HIV and malaria are reported. Studies are contradictory about the frequency and severity of malaria in HIV infected people. Malaria does not appear to act as a classic opportunist in immune compromised hosts. People who have grown up in endemic regions often retain partial immunity to malaria, and there is no solid evidence that this immunity is lost as HIV disease progresses.

Malaria Treatment in HIV

A study in Malawi reported a lowering of plasma HIV levels during SP treatment of acute falciparum malaria. At baseline, 47 HIV positive men and women with confirmed symptomatic falciparum malaria had a median viral load of 151,000 copies/mL. The baseline median viral load of the control group, consisting of 42 asymptomatic, aparasitic HIV positive men and women, was 22,000 copies/mL. Twenty seven malaria subjects and 22 non malaria subjects completed four weeks of follow-up. After four weeks on treatment, the median viral load of the 27 malaria patients had declined from 191,000 to 120,000 copies/mL. The median viral load of the control group increased slightly. (Hoffman)

A different anti-malarial agent is chloroquine, a drug with immune modulatory qualities that has also been reported to have an inhibitory effect on HIV in vitro – Pardridge; Savarino. Although conducted before the availability of sensitive viral load assays, a clinical trial that compared chloroquine to AZT in asymptomatic patients reported equivalent reductions in recoverable HIV after 16 weeks – Sperber. A study in Uganda reported no difference between the incidence (but not the severity) of malarial episodes in children with or without HIV. The authors wondered whether the anti-HIV properties of the chloroquine administered to both groups had confounded their observations—Kalyesubula. Compounds related to chloroquine are currently being investigated as HIV integrase inhibitors—Mathe.

Drug resistant strains of malaria are threatening to cripple efforts to arrest the epidemic. Chloroquine resistant Plasmodium is widespread in many parts of Southeast Asia and increasingly common in Africa. Resistance to SP has been noted in Tanzania and elsewhere. Chloroquine and SP, as first and second line treatments, once offered a cure for about twenty cents per person. The drugs needed to treat resistant strains of malaria cost many times that amount and will not be widely available in poor countries. As with tuberculosis and HIV, the solution to effective treatment of this resistance prone pathogen may lie in adopting combination therapy with agents that block the Plasmodium life cycle at two crucial points instead of one, thereby multiplying protection against resistance—White.

Although expensive HIV drugs are not likely to become available soon for everyday treatment in malarial regions, the efficacy of low cost, short course antiretroviral therapy to prevent mother to child transmission during birth has been established. The use of AZT and nevirapine in pregnancy is growing and could soon become standard of care throughout most of the world. Although pregnant women in endemic malarial regions are routinely prescribed prophylaxis for malaria, no studies have been made of the potential for pharmacologic, toxic and teratologic interactions between these various classes of drugs—Okereke.

The Immunological Connection

The mechanisms used by the immune system to fight malaria are not fully understood, although it is clear that both humoral and cell mediated immunity are involved and that various T-cell subsets are important for regulating the immune response—Troye-Blomberg. HIV too has an intricate relationship with the immune system, and it appears that there may be several points of intersection between the pathogenesis and response to each disease.

Some have suggested that the malarial antigens and pigments released during the burst of red blood cells stimulate cytokines that can activate HIV replication. The investigators in Malawi who noted lower HIV levels in people treated with SP also measured levels of tumor necrosis factor (TNF alpha), a cellular signaling protein or cytokine that has been associated with increased rates of HIV replication. TNF alpha is released in response to anti-malarial immune activation. But during SP malaria treatment, blood levels of TNF alpha decreased. This adds weight to the suggestion that suppressing malarial infection may result in a lowered HIV viral burden–Hoffman.

Different clinical manifestations of malaria are associated with different states of immune dysregulation. In Ghana, children with cerebral malaria had significantly higher levels of TNF, TNF receptors, and IL-10 (another cellular signaling cytokine) than did those with severe malarial anemia or uncomplicated malaria—Akanmori.

This picture is further complicated by reports that various common malaria treatments such as quinine and artesunate directly affect TNF levels in vitro—Ittarat.

Another cytokine that increases during acute malaria is granulocyte colony stimulating factor (G-CSF)—Stoiser. G-CSF stimulates the production of neutrophils (white blood cells that help fight bacterial and fungal infections). A clinical trial of G-CSF versus placebo in AIDS patients reported a significantly lower incidence of bacterial infections for those receiving G-CSF but no difference in HIV viral load—Kuritzkes.

A connection between HIV and malaria may exist in the way the immune system responds to certain similar molecular features on their structural proteins. An analysis using Western blot antibody diagnostics found overlapping immune reactivity in blood containing HIV antigens and that with P. falciparum antigens. HIV negative subjects from Papua, New Guinea, an endemic malarial region, reacted positively to certain HIV antigens. Similarly, blood from HIV positive persons from non malarious regions reacted positively in immunoblot tests for antibodies to P. falciparum antigen—Elm.

If HIV infection stimulates an immune response to P. falciparum, it may help explain unexpected findings of decreased malaria mortality in a group of HIV positive children. Of 121 children with HIV entering a clinic in Kinshasa, Zaire, 41 had malaria. Half of the malaria cases were moderate to severe, and all cases were treated with quinine. None of the 41 children with HIV and malaria died compared to 25 of the 71 children with just HIV. While no one died in the coinfected pediatric population, there was a 14% death rate among HIV negative children with malaria. The prevalence of malaria at this hospital was the same for children with or without HIV—Dayachi. These results seem to be contradicted by a later Ugandan study finding that pediatric malaria patients with HIV had more hospitalizations and required more transfusions than those without HIV—Kalyesubula.

Others have proposed that the immune response to malaria can increase the pool of lymphocytes available for HIV infection, resulting in accelerated progression to AIDS. Whether this actually occurs is not known. Much research still needs to be done to understand the interactions between the immune system and these all too common pathogens.

Malaria as Opportunistic Infection in HIV

As HIV spreads, it interacts with other infectious diseases, facilitated by the increase in numbers of immunosuppressed individuals and because its own clinical course can be altered by other infections. Infectious diseases often 'synergize', or negatively affect each other, and this is most noticeable with HIV and tuberculosis (TB). In areas of high HIV prevalence, the incidence of TB infection is increased, with a resultant increase in mortality. In addition, susceptibility to HIV can be increased by other infections, notably sexually transmitted infections (STIs), leading to high rates of HIV transmission in communities with high prevalence of STIs.

In Africa, the HIV pandemic has been superimposed on the longstanding malaria pandemic, where P. falciparum malaria is consistently one of the major causes of infant and child mortality. The high prevalence of both HIV and malaria infection in Africa means that even small interactions between the two could have substantial effects on populations.

With the inception of the Roll Back Malaria partnership in 1998, there was recognition that previous gradual declines in malaria mortality had been reversed during the 1990's, and that interactions between malaria and HIV could be one contributor.

Early research did not indicate any direct, biological association between HIV and malaria, although it was noted that malaria associated anaemia treated with unscreened blood transfusions contributed to HIV transmission. In more recent years, three key issues have focussed much of the research effort:

1. Does HIV/AIDS increase susceptibility to malaria infection or increase severity of acute malarial episodes?
2. Does malaria infection accelerate progression of HIV/AIDS?

3. What is the impact of malaria and HIV co-infection during pregnancy?

Effect of HIV on Malaria

HIV infection increases the incidence and severity of clinical malaria. In non pregnant adults, HIV infection has been found to roughly double the risk of malaria parasitemia and clinical malaria. In east and southern Africa, where HIV prevalence is near 30%, it is estimated that about one-quarter to one-third of clinical malaria in adults (including during pregnancy) can be accounted for by HIV. Little research has been carried out in children, although anaemia from multiple causes is common and associated with increased mortality in HIV infected children.

Effect of malaria on HIV

Although the effect of malaria on HIV has not been so well documented, some recent research is now adding to the growing body of evidence. Acute malaria infection increases viral load, and one study found that this increased viral load was reversed by effective malaria treatment. This malaria associated increase in viral load could lead to increased transmission of HIV and more rapid disease progression, with substantial public health implications.

One recent study found that daily cotrimoxazole prophylaxis among HIV infected adults reduced malaria incidence by 80% in Uganda. Although this effect would be expected to vary, depending on epidemiological setting and patterns of drug resistance, it may be relevant for both pregnant women and adults more generally.

Technical Issues

- If the transient elevation in viral load associated with malaria infection can be reversed with effective malaria treatment (as shown by prospective studies), malaria prevention and control may prove to be beneficial in reducing HIV transmission and slowing progression to AIDS.

- Large-scale use of trimethoprim sulfamethoxazole (cotrimoxazole) for prophylaxis of opportunistic infections in HIV positive patients, although of possible benefit in reducing the incidence of malaria, may also increase drug pressure for other antifolate combinations. This may potentially accelerate resistance to sulfadoxine pyrimethamine (SP), which is being increasingly used for the treatment of acute uncomplicated malaria in Africa and antenatal IPT programmes. Conversely, expanding use of SP in Africa might further lead to the development of resistance to cotrimoxazole by other pathogens, such as Streptococcus pneumoniae. The effectiveness of both of these drugs needs to be carefully monitored in country programmes.

- It is estimated that 5%-10% of new HIV infections are caused by unsafe blood products. This has enormous implications for the management of severe anemia, including that which occurs during childhood as a result of severe malaria infection (see below).

Chapter 7

Investigations

ROUTINE LABORATORY DIAGNOSIS

There are many methods to detect malaria parasites which are implemented according to the facilities available at a given place.

Direct Parasite Demonstration

Thick Blood Film

Test is done by counting the number of parasites present in 200 WBC and multiplying the parasites counted by 40. This will give the parasite count per micro liter of blood. The most accurate counts are obtained by counting the total parasites seen in a given measured volume of blood.

Advantage of the thick blood film is that it can give the total number of parasites in the blood.

Disadvantage of the thick blood film is the lysis of the RBCs during the staining process, making the slide more difficult to read with the absence of RBC features and irregularities in the thickness of the film.

Thin Blood Film

Advantage of thin film is that because of the fixed monolayer of red blood cells, the morphological identification of the parasite is easier to see and count. The ability to count parasites in sequential blood films enables the response to therapy to be monitored specially for P. falciparum.

Test is done by counting the number of parasitized RBC seen in 10,000 Red Blood Cells.

Disadvantage of thin film is that this helps in diagnosing malaria when the malaria is not endemic and parasites in blood are less.

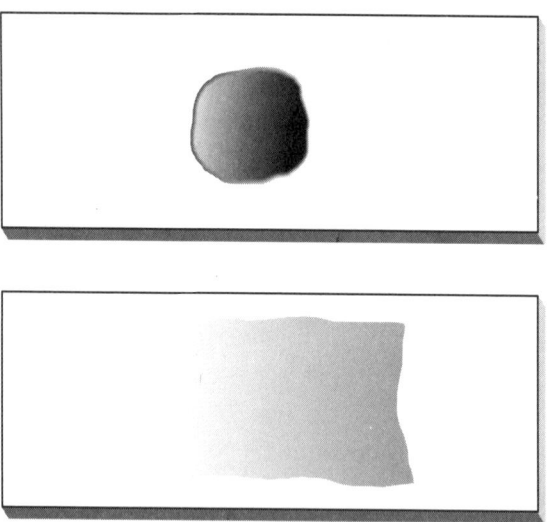

QBC Method

A special glass capillary tube is filled with 20 µl blood. The inner side of this tube is coated with anticoagulants and the dye acridine orange. Afterwards the tube is centrifuged (10,000 g x 5 minutes).

The blood cells are thus separated according to density. The buffy coat is the part of the centrifuged blood which contains platelets and white blood cells. In the tube is a longitudinal plastic float with the same density as the buffy coat. The float serves to spread the buffy coat and adjacent cells and press them in a thin layer against the wall. Since parasitized red blood cells are lighter than non parasitized ones and heavier than white blood cells, infected red blood cells will be found on top of the red cell column, just below the white blood cells, right against the buffy coat. The parasites in this layer can be observed using a fluorescence microscope.

Advantage of this technique is that the readings of this test are much quicker than reading thick or thin smears.

It is used in hospitals where many samples are tested daily.

Disadvantage of this test is that it requires training and appropriate apparatus. This test cannot identify the species of the parasite. Wide inter-observer variability. The specially prepared disposable tubes need to be available as well as a microhaematocrit centrifuge and a microscope with a UV lens. This test helps in differentiating malaria with other diseases like:-

Filariasis

Babesiosis

Trypanosomiasis (Chagas disease, Sleeping Sickness)

Relapsing Fever (Borreliosis)

Basic principle lies in the fluoro chrome staining of plasmodial nucleic acid (sensitivity 42-94%) differentiating species to a fairly well (specificity P.vivax 52%, P. falciparum 93%).

Indirect Demonstration of Parasite Exposure

Antibody based methods

1. IFAT
2. ELISA

Antigen Detection Test

This consists of two tests:

1. Histidien rich protein-2 (HRP-2) for P. falciparum. It is a dipstick test which yields results within 10 minutes and has a specificity of 90%.

2. pLDH test which can detect any plasmodial species and which also is a dipstick based test. It has comparable specificity and sensitivity.

RAPID DIAGNOSTIC TEST

Malaria rapid diagnostic test assists in the diagnosis of malaria by providing evidence of the presence of malarial parasites in human blood. These tests are an alternative to diagnosis based on clinical grounds or microscopy, particularly where good quality microscopy services cannot be readily provided.

Rapid diagnostic tests or RDTs, for malaria offer the potential to extend accurate diagnosis of malaria to areas when microscopy services are not available such as in remote locations or after regular laboratory hours. Rapid malaria diagnostic tests have been developed in the lateral flow format. These tests use finger stick or venous blood, take only 10 to 15 minutes, and do not require a laboratory. Even non clinical staff can easily learn to perform the test and interpret the results.

Malaria RDTs rely on the detection of parasite specific antigens (proteins) circulating in the bloodstream.

Some malaria treatment programs require testing of patients after treatment to confirm that parasites have been cleared.

ELISA TEST

This test measures past evidences of malarial fever.

POLYMERASE CHAIN REACTIONS

PCR test is the test to identify the amino acid sequence in a polypeptide chain of a specific protein. In travelers returning to developed countries, this test is effective for detecting all four species of malaria. The PCR test has also been found useful in undiagnosed fever, when is not diagnosed symptomatologically.

DETECTION OF ANTIMALARIAL ANTIBODIES

Malaria antibody detection is performed using the indirect fluorescent antibody (IFA) test. The IFA procedure can be used to determine if a patient has been infected with Plasmodium. Because of the time required for development of antibody and also the persistence of antibodies, serologic testing is not practical for routine diagnosis of acute malaria.

Antibody detection may be useful for:

1. Screening blood donors involved in cases of transfusion induced malaria when the donor's parasitemia may be below the detectable level of blood film examination.
2. Testing a patient with a febrile illness who is suspected of having malaria and from whom repeated blood smears are negative.
3. Testing a patient who has been recently treated for malaria but in whom the diagnosis is questioned.
4. Species specific testing is available for the four human species, P. falciparum, P. vivax, P. malariae and P. ovale.

5. Enzyme immunoassays have also been employed as a tool to screen blood donors, but have limited sensitivity due to the use of only Plasmodium falciparum antigen instead of antigens of all four human species.

INTRALEUCOCYTIC MALARIA PIGMENT

Intraleucocytic malaria pigment has been suggested as a measure of disease severity in malaria.

FLOW CYTOMETRY

Flowcytometry and automated hematology analyzers is useful in diagnosis of malaria during routine blood counts. In cases of malaria, abnormal cell clusters and small particles with DNA fluorescence, probably free malarial parasites, have been seen on automated hematology analyzers and it is suggested that malaria can be suspected based on the scatter plots produced on the analyzer.

Automated detection of malaria pigment in white blood cells may also suggest a possibility of malaria with a sensitivity of 95% and specificity of 88%.

MASS SPECTROMETRY

In vitro detection of the malarial parasite at a sensitivity of 10 parasites/µL of blood.

Chapter 8

Prevention of Malaria

Malaria cannot be eradicated but the transmission can be prevented. This requires co-operation at all levels.

A plan to fight malaria is to be done at three levels:

1. Individual level
2. Community level
3. Government level

INDIVIDUAL LEVEL

Measures that an individual can take are as follows:

Use of mosquito repellent creams, liquids, coils, mats and the like.

Screening of the houses with wire mesh

Use of bed nets treated with insecticides

For optimal prevention of malaria, protection from mosquito bites is essential, even if you are taking preventive medicines.

Avoid Mosquito Bites

Mosquito bites particularly at twilight and at night, so you should take most precautions during this time.

Sleep in rooms that are properly screened with gauze over the windows and doors. There should be no holes in the gauze and no unscreened entry points to the room. Air conditioned rooms are good, too.

Spray the room with an insecticide before entering to kill any mosquitoes that have got inside during the day. Otherwise, you should use a mosquito net around your bed, impregnated with an insecticide such as pyrethrum or permethrin.

Long trousers, long sleeved clothing and socks thick enough to stop the mosquitoes biting will also protect you, and should be worn outside after sunset. However, it may be hard to follow such advice in a hot climate. Light colors are less attractive to mosquitoes.

Use Mosquito Repellent Cream

Mosquito repellent containing diethyl toluamide (DEET) is recommended as the most effective form of bite preventive treatment. It has an excellent safety profile in adults, children and pregnant women.

It's important that the manufacturer's recommendations are not exceeded, particularly when using it on small children. Insect repellents containing over 30 per cent DEET will effectively repel mosquitoes when applied to exposed skin.

Lemon scent was found to protect citrus groves from mosquitoes, and refined lemon eucalyptus oil on skin also repels mosquitoes.

Mosquito Nets

When sleeping outdoors or in an unscreened room, have an insecticide treated mosquito net around your bed. This significantly reduces the risk of bites.

The net should be small meshed, with no holes, and tucked in under the bottom sheet. During the day, it should be rolled up, so mosquitoes and other insects can't get inside while it's not in use.

Take your own net with you. You can't always expect to find an impregnated net at your destination.

Impregnation lasts from six months to one year, depending on how much the net is used and whether you pack it away in a plastic bag when you return from the tropics. Just remember not to wash the net in between reimpregnation with the insecticide.

Preventive Medicines

Taking medicines to prevent malaria is essential if you are visiting an area where malaria is prevalent. The problem can be choosing the most appropriate antimalarial for the country you're visiting. Because resistance to chloroquine and other drugs is spreading, preventive medicines that were effective five years ago may no longer be so.

The geographic spread of chloroquine resistance in the malarial parasite Plasmodium falciparum is increasing. It exists throughout sub-Saharan Africa, Southeast Asia, the Indian subcontinent and large portions of South America.

There are currently six drugs on the market that are licensed for preventing malaria, and the most appropriate one(s) will depend on the country you are visiting and your individual circumstances.

COMMUNITY LEVEL

Community Participation

Sensitizing and involving the community for detection of anopheles mosquito breeding places and their elimination.

Collaboration with business chambers.

Schemes involving Non Governmental Organizations in programme strategies.

GOVERNMENT LEVEL

National Anti Malaria Programme

Malaria is a common disease of the tropical world caused by the parasite Plasmodium. The disease is transmitted from man to man by the infective bites of female mosquitoes belonging to the genus anopheles, as the mouth parts of male mosquitoes are not developed for biting and cannot pierce the skin. There are 4 species of malarial parasites, of which 3 species are found in India. These are:

P. vivax that may cause relapse of malaria but seldom death.

P. falciparum that causes malignant malaria and may lead to death.

P. malariae that may cause severe malaria, small numbers found in foothills in Orissa.

P. ovale not found in India.

Often 0.5% to 2% of P. falciparum cases (malignant variety of malaria) may develop severe malaria with complications. In such cases death rates may be 30% or more, if timely treatment is not commenced. All malaria mortality in India is due to P. falciparum only.

The disease manifests with sudden onset of high fever with rigors and sensation of extreme cold followed by feeling of burning heat, leading to profuse sweating and remission of fever by crisis thereafter. The febrile paroxysms occur every alternate day. Headache, body ache, nausea, etc. may be associated features. However in atypical cases, classical presentation may not manifest. Since infection of any kind leads to fever, the strategy adopted by NAMP is to test all fever cases for malaria in a laboratory under the microscope. This practice ensures that malaria among the fever cases are not missed, and those found positive for malaria are given full course of malaria treatment. On an average NAMP examines 80-90 million fever cases, and the current malaria incidence is about 2 million cases annually.

Malaria transmission occurs in almost all areas of India except areas above 1800 metres sea level. The country's 95% population lives in malaria risk areas. Malaria in India is unevenly distributed. In most parts of the country about 90% malaria is unstable with relatively low incidence but with a risk of increase in cases in epidemic form every 7 to 10 or more years. This depends on the immune status of the population and the breeding potential of the mosquitoes, rainfall being the leading cause of malaria epidemics as it creates high mosquito population. In north-eastern states efficient malaria transmission is maintained during most months of the year. Intermediate level of stability of malaria transmission is maintained in the plains of India in the forests and forest fringes, predominantly tribal settlements in eight states (Andhra Pradesh, Jharkhand, Gujarat, Madhya Pradesh, Chhatisgarh, Maharashtra, Orissa and Rajasthan).

National Programme for Control of Malaria

At the time of independence, malaria was responsible for an estimated 75 million cases and 0.8 million deaths annually. The

Government of India launched the National Malaria Control Programme (NMCP) in 1953. DDT spraying resulted in a sharp decline in malaria in all areas under spray. In 1958, GOI converted NMCP to the National Malaria Eradication Programme (NMEP). The strategy of malaria eradication was highly successful and the cases were reduced to about 100,000 and deaths due to malaria were eliminated by 1965-66. Subsequently the programme faced various technical obstacles and financial and administrative constraints, which led to countrywide increase in the number of cases. 6.47 million malaria cases were reported in 1976, the highest since resurgence. In 1977 the Modified Plan of Operation (MPO) was launched with the immediate objectives to prevent deaths and to reduce morbidity due to malaria. The programme was integrated with primary health care delivery system. Selective indoor residual spray by stratifying areas based on cases per 1,000 populations in a year i.e. the Annual Parasite Incidence (API) of 2 and above was recommended in the MPO. Malaria incidence declined to about 2 million cases by the year 2000 and thereafter.

Enhanced Malaria Control Project (EMCP)

The states of Andhra Pradesh, Chattisgarh, Gujarat, Jharkhand, Madhya Pradesh, Maharashtra, Rajasthan and Orissa together contribute around 60-70% cases and deaths due to malaria. World Bank assisted Enhanced Malaria Control Project is in operation in 1045 malaria hardcore tribal PHCs of 100 districts covering 62 million populations in these states. Nineteen towns of 10 States have also been included under EMCP. In these areas, attempts are being made to have an integrated strategy for malaria control which includes providing for presumptive treatment to fever cases at each village; presumptive radical treatment at health facilities in high risk areas; promotion of use of insecticide treated bed nets; use of larvivorous fish in mosquito breeding sites and selective indoor residual spray in high risk areas. The project period has been extended for a period of one year i.e. up to 31st March 2004.

Urban Malaria Scheme (UMS)

Since the resurgence of malaria in early 1970s, urban malaria has been recognized as an important problem contributing to overall malaria morbidity in the country. To assist the states in control of malaria in urban areas, Urban Malaria Scheme (UMS) was launched in 1971. The scheme is being implemented in 131 towns in the country. Urban malaria poses problems because of haphazard expansion of urban areas. The urban malaria vector, anopheles stephensi breeds in stored water and domestic containers. Construction activities and aggregation of labour provide ideal opportunities for vector to breed and transmit malaria in urban areas.

Under UMS, the centre provides assistance in kind which includes larvicide and 2% pyrethrum extract. The operational cost and the cost of MLO and equipment are borne by the states. However, the centre bears the operational cost as well as material and equipment for UMS in the north-eastern states and Chandigarh.

Current Malaria Control Strategies

The main control strategies under the programme are:

Early Case Detection and Prompt Treatment (EDPT) to provide relief to the patient, and reduce reservoir of the infection.

Selective Vector Control by appropriate insecticidal spray in rural areas and recurrent anti-larval measures including biological methods like use of larvivorous fish.

Promotion of personal prophylactic measures including use of Insecticide Treated Mosquito Nets (ITMN), etc., and promotion of bioenvironmental control measures.

Capacity building of optimal utilization of the technical manpower for the programme.

Chapter 9

Control of Vector

Following methods are adopted for vector control:
1. Use of indoor residual spray with insecticides recommended
2. Use of chemical larvicides like Abate in portable water
3. Aerosol space spray during daytime
4. Malathion fogging during outbreaks
5. Malaria can be prevented only by two most important strategies and these are
    i. Early detection
    ii. Prompt treatment

STRATEGIES FOR VECTOR CONTROL

1. Effectiveness in terms of technical and economical aspects.
2. Community involvement/ partnership.
3. Combine with chemotherapy treatment.
4. Expanding the application of insecticide treated bed nets.

5. Indication of residual spraying where necessary.
6. Additional application of other environmental measures for mosquito control.
7. The main vector control measures are sleeping inside the bed nets and insecticide treated bed net.
8. In remote and border areas, bed nets are subsidized for poor people.

VECTOR CONTROL MEASURES

1. Insecticide treated bed nets (ITNs)
2. Indoor Residual Spraying (IRS) with insecticides
3. Environmental Management and Modification
4. Seeding of stream
5. Stream clearing
6. Personal protection
7. Chemo-prophylaxis
8. Mosquito repellant
9. Insecticide
10. Selection of insecticide based on evaluation done according to distribution of vectors and impact on disease and community
11. Insecticide had been specified and considered by WHO
12. Residual effectiveness enough for operation one round per year
13. Safety and Cost effectivenesses

Insecticides used are:

i. Lambdacyhalothrin

    a. ICON 10 WP for spraying ($32mg/m2$, effect in 9-11months)

    b. ICON 2,5 CS for bed net impregnation (20mg/m2, effect in 7-11months)

ii. Alphacypermethrin

    a. Fendona 10 CS for both spraying (30mg/m2, effect in 9-10 months) and bed net impregnation (25mg/m2, effect in 6-10months).

    b. Permethrin 50EC (before 2001) for bed net impregnation (2mg/m2, effect in 5-7 months)

MALARIA ZONES IDENTIFICATION AND MANAGEMENT

Highly Endemic

A zone where there are more than 10 cases per 1000 population in a year.

Treatment and Management

1. Spraying extensively to kill larvae and mosquitoes.
2. The drugs should be highly effective.
3. Each person should have a treated bed net.
4. Proper surveillance is must.
5. The primary, secondary and tertiary health services should be available, for proper management of the case.

Moderately Endemic

A zone where there are between 5-10 cases per 1000 population in a year.

Treatment and Management

1. Management of migration.
2. Proper surveillance is must.

3. Each person should have a treated bed net.
4. The primary, secondary and tertiary health services should be available, for proper management of the case.

Low Endemic

A zone where there are more than 5 cases per 1000 population in a year.

Treatment and Management

1. Spraying where people do not use bed net.
2. Proper surveillance is must.

Free from Malaria

A zone where there have been no indigenous cases in 5 years.

Treatment and Management

1. Management of migration population and the cases.
2. A proper provision of the drugs and bed nets.

No Malaria Transmission

A zone where there is no indigenous case.

Treatment and Management

1. Management of migration population and the cases.
2. A proper provision of the drugs and bed nets.
3. Bed nets to be given to people who are going to malaria area.

Chapter 10

Travel Precautions

Malaria is often transmitted to humans through a bite by an infected mosquito, particularly the female anopheles mosquito, known as a dusk to dawn biter. The infection is also transmitted through blood transfusion with infected blood, or with a shared needle. A mother could also pass the infection to her unborn child.

Malaria is a constant feature of Sub-Saharan Africa, Middle East, South Asia, south-east Asia, Oceania, Haiti, Central and South America, some parts of Dominican Republic, Mexico, and North Africa.

In India, the states which are most affected by malaria are Orissa, Assam, Madhya Pradesh, Jharkhand, Gujarat, Himachal Pradesh, Arunachal Pradesh, Uttar Pradesh and Bihar.

1. Antimalarial drugs are to be taken under the guidance of physician only.

   Antimalarial drugs include atovaquone/proguanil, doxycycline and mefloquine.

2. Take precautions like staying inside as much as possible during those times. If staying outdoor, make sure that you wear a long-sleeve shirt, pants and even a hat. Always apply insect repellent to the exposed skin.

3. Malaria can be very fatal. If one develops a fever or flu like symptoms then one should try to take any anti-pyretic drug. But should seek medical advice as soon as possible.
4. When travelling with kids to malaria risk places, get your children vaccinated 4-6 weeks before the travel. Each age has a specific dosage, so take time to let the pharmacy fill your children's prescription.

Malaria in humans is caused by one of the four protozoan species of the genus Plasmodium, P. falciparum, P. vivax, P. ovale, or P. malariae. All species are transmitted by the bite of an infected female anopheles mosquito. Occasionally, transmission occurs by blood transfusion, organ transplantation, needle sharing, or congenitally from mother to foetus.

Malaria is characterized by fever and influenza like symptoms, including chills, headache, myalgias, and malaise; these symptoms can occur at intervals. Malaria may be associated with anemia and jaundice, and P. falciparum infections can cause seizures, mental confusion, kidney failure, coma, and death. Taking proper precautions can control the disease.

Malaria symptoms can develop as early as 7 days after initial exposure in a malaria endemic area and as late as several months after departure from a malarious area or after chemoprophylaxis treatment has been terminated. The estimated risk for a traveller acquiring malaria depends on the following aspects:

1. Region to be visited
2. Time and type of travel
3. Intensity of transmission

RISK FOR TRAVELLERS

All travellers going to malaria endemic countries, even for

short periods of time may be at risk for becoming infected with malaria.

The persons residing in malarious endemic area are not allowed to donate blood for three years after leaving their area of residence.

Persons who have had malaria are not allowed to donate blood for 3 years after treatment for malaria.

Adventure travellers are usually more exposed to malaria than ordinary travellers due to the nature of their activities and the fact that they travel to the more remote locations.

No vaccine is currently available. Only taking an appropriate drug regimen and using anti mosquito measures will help prevent malaria.

There is no method to protect completely against the risk for contracting malaria.

The mosquitoes bite at night time i.e. between dusk and dawn, hence it is advised to take protective measures to reduce contact with mosquitoes, especially during these hours. Measures to avoid mosquito bites are:

1. Staying in well screened areas.
2. By using mosquito bed nets.
3. By wearing clothes that cover most of the body.
4. By using insect repellent for use if one is in open area, like DEET.

(N, N-diethylmetatoluamide), DEET formulations as high as 50% are recommended for both adults and children older than 2 months of age.

5. By using an insect spray in living and sleeping areas during evening and nighttime hours.
6. By sleeping under insecticide treated bed nets.

Commonly advised sprays or insecticides are:

i. Permethrin (Permanone) is available as a liquid or spray
ii. Deltamethrin

Drugs used in treatment and active against the parasite forms in the blood are:

i. Chloroquine
ii. Sulfadoxine-pyrimethamine (Fansidar®)
iii. Mefloquine (Lariam®)

Stages in the plasmodium life cycle when anti-malarial drugs act

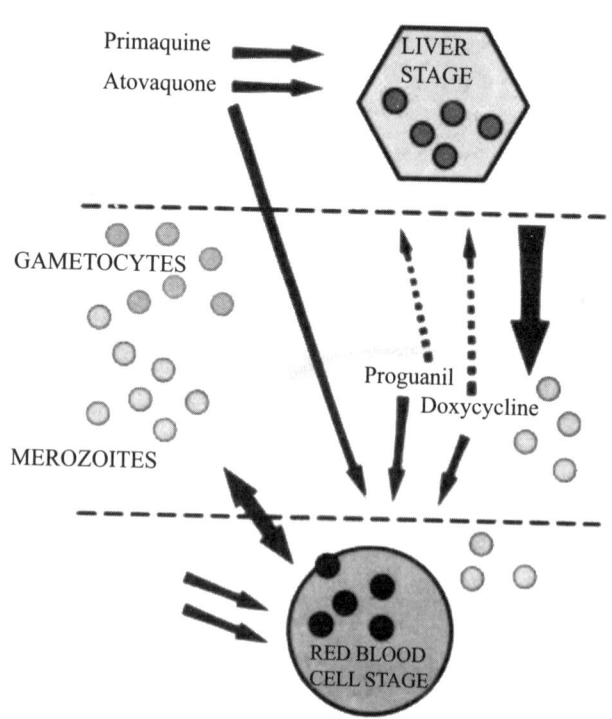

iv. Atovaquone-proguanil (Malarone®)

v. Quinine

vi. Doxycycline

vii. Artemisin derivatives

The Different Drug Regimens

Regimen 1

Mefloquine one 250mg tablet weekly, OR

Doxycycline one 100mg capsule daily, OR

Malarone one tablet daily.

Regimen 2

Chloroquine 300mg weekly (2x150mg tablets), PLUS

Proguanil 200mg daily (2x100mg tablets).

Regimen 3

Chloroquine 300mg weekly (2x150mg tablets) OR

Proguanil 200mg daily (2x100mg tablets).

Regimen 4

No prophylactic tablets required but anti mosquito measures should be strictly observed. Avoid mosquito bites by covering up with clothing such as long sleeves and long trousers especially after sunset, using insect repellents on exposed skin and when necessary, sleeping under a mosquito net.

Proguanil : 100mg tablets are supplied as Paludrine Tablets.

Chloroquine : 150mg tablets are supplied as Nivaquine or Avloclor Tablets.

Mefloquine : 250mg tablets are supplied as Lariam Tablets.

Malarone : It is a combination of Atovaquone 250mg and Proguanil 100mg

LENGTH OF PROPHYLAXIS

1. Chloroquine, Proguanil and Maloprim

    Start one week before travel, throughout your stay in an endemic area and continue for four weeks after return.

2. Mefloquine (Lariam)

    Start two and a half weeks before travel, throughout your stay in an endemic area and continue for four weeks after return.

3. Doxycycline

    Start two days before travel, throughout your stay in an endemic area and continue for four weeks after return.

4. Malarone

    Start two days before travel, throughout your stay in an endemic area and continue for one week after return.

Important! Take the tablets Absolutely Regularly, Preferably with or After a Meal

Long Term Use of Anti-Malaria Drugs

1. Chloroquine: May be taken for time period exceeding five years.
2. Paludrine: May be taken for time period exceeding five years.
3. Maloprim: Can be taken for time period up to one year.
4. Mefloquine: Can be taken for time period up to one year.
5. Doxycycline: Can be taken for time period up to six months.
6. Malarone: Can be used for travel time period up to one year.

Chloroquine or Nivaquine, Avloclor

Is taken weekly and is the preferred drug for the few areas without chloroquine resistance. It is used in combination with proguanil in areas with a slightly higher risk of chloroquine resistant malaria.

Chloroquine can be used on its own or in combination with other anti-malarial drugs to increase its effectiveness.

Side effects of Chloroquine are bone marrow suppression, loss of hair, damage to the retina and some dysfunction of the brain. It may exacerbate psoriasis in the patient.

It should be used with caution in pregnancy.

Chloroquine was successful in combating the disease during the 1950s, but the malaria parasite became resistant to the drug.

Proguanil or Paludrine

Proguanil or Paludrine is taken daily, and is an alternative to chloroquine in areas without chloroquine resistance. Resistance to proguanil has also developed over the years.

The combination of chloroquine and proguanil was about 70 per cent effective in Africa 10 years ago, but is much less than this now in much of Africa (mainly south of the Sahara).

However, it is still the recommended combination for the Indian subcontinent and various other low risk parts of the world. Both drugs should be started one week before travel and continued for a further four weeks after leaving the malarious area.

Mefloquine (Lariam)

Mefloquine has the worst known side effects of all malaria drugs.

It is contraindicated for people who suffer from depression, anxiety, or other psychiatric disturbances.

Side effects: It causes psychological disturbances, hallucinations, psychosis, seizures, depression and also hair loss.

Mefloquine is not recommended during pregnancy or breast-feeding because it is secreted in breast milk.

Other milder side effects include sleep disturbances and abnormal dreams. It is taken weekly and should be started two to three weeks before traveling, so that three doses have been taken before departure. This enables blood levels of the drug to reach a protective level.

More than 75 per cent of side effects will have appeared in this time if they are going to happen, allowing time to change to another antimalarial drug, if necessary.

Mefloquine should be continued for four weeks after leaving the malarious area. It should not be taken by people with a history of psychiatric disturbances (including depression) or convulsions (e.g. epilepsy).

Doxycyline or Malarone

Doxycyline or Malarone are considered to be the drugs of first choice in areas where the malaria is mefloquine resistant. They are also an alternative to mefloquine in areas of high chloroquine resistance.

Doxycyline and Malarone (Doxycycline, eg Vibramycin) is considered to be as effective as mefloquine. It is taken daily, starting one to two days before travel and continuing for four weeks after leaving the malarious area.

People who take doxycycline should be aware that it may make their skin very sensitive to the sun and women may be more prone to thrush.

Malarone (containing proguanil and atovaquone) is also considered to be of similar effectiveness as mefloquine. It is only licensed to prevent Plasmodium falciparum malaria (the malignant type, which is often resistant to other antimalarials).

It is not licensed for longer than 28 days of use and so may be useful for brief visits to high risk areas.

It is taken daily and should be taken with a meal rich in fats (eg yoghurt) or a milky drink to avoid the risk of it not being adequately absorbed from the stomach.

It should be started two to three days before travel and only needs to be continued for a week after leaving the malarious area.

Chloroquine and proguanil are the only antimalarial drugs that can be bought from your pharmacist without a prescription, the others are only available from your doctor.

Whatever preventive medicines are used, it's important they are taken regularly and as directed by your doctor or pharmacist, while you are away and when you return.

The risk of malaria increases with the length of stay, so it is important to keep taking your preventive medicines throughout a long visit. Most deaths from malaria occur in those who take their preventive medicines irregularly, or not at all.

If you decide to go anyway, or if you are obliged to go, extra care should be taken to protect small children, because they get very ill very quickly if falciparum malaria is involved.

Medicines for Children

Preventive medicines should be given to breastfed as well as bottle fed babies because they are not protected by the mother's medicine passing into the breast milk.

Chloroquine and proguanil may be given safely to babies and young children, but the doses used are much smaller than those recommended for adults. It is very important to check with your pharmacist or doctor regarding the correct doses for children aged 12 years or under.

Mefloquine may be given from three months onwards. There is little experience with this medicine in children under three months or weighing less than 5kg and it is not recommended in these cases.

Doxycycline should not be given to children under 12 years of age.

Malarone should not be given to children weighing less than 40kg. Malarone Paediatric, can be given to children weighing between 11kg and 40kg, but should not be given to children weighing below 11kg.

For administration, antimalarial medicines may be crushed and mixed with jam, banana, or similar foods. Syrup formulations are available for certain medicines, but have shorter shelf lives in tropical areas.

Remember to keep all antimalarial medicines in childproof containers out of children's reach. Chloroquine can be fatal to children if the recommended dose is exceeded.

PREGNANCY AND BREASTFEEDING

Pregnant women are discouraged by the World Health Organization from travelling to malarious regions where there is chloroquine resistant falciparum malaria, because malaria increases the risk of abortion, premature birth, still birth and maternal death.

Just as for children, an extra effort should be made to protect yourself from mosquitoes and malaria if you are obliged to travel.

If you are planning to travel to a malarious region or have any other travel vaccines, it is very important that you tell your doctor if you are pregnant or planning to become pregnant.

Medicines for Pregnant Women

Both chloroquine and proguanil have no special risk for pregnant women, and should be administered together. Pregnant women who use proguanil should also take a daily folic acid supplement.

In countries where resistance to chloroquine and proguanil is high, it may be necessary for your doctor to prescribe mefloquine. There is evidence that mefloquine may be associated with an increased risk of stillbirths, so it should only be used during pregnancy if the need for it is great.

The decision to prescribe mefloquine is made after weighing up the benefits of preventing malaria, versus the risks of harmful effects on the foetus and the risk of contracting the disease.

In scenarios where other medicines are not effective, the benefits of using mefloquine may outweigh the risks, but your doctor would need to decide this in conjunction with you. If pregnant women accidentally take mefloquine during pregnancy, there is no reason to terminate the pregnancy.

Malarone should be avoided unless there is no suitable alternative. Pregnant women who use Malarone should also take a daily folic acid supplement.

Doxycycline should not be taken by pregnant women.

Medicines for Breastfeeding Mothers

Breastfeeding mothers can safely take chloroquine and proguanil. However not enough of these medicines passes into the breast milk to provide protection for the child.

Mefloquine, doxycycline and malarone should not be taken by breastfeeding mothers.

Most people living in malaria prevalent areas have acquired some immunity to the disease.

Visitors will not have immunity, and will need to take preventive medications and even pregnant women should take preventive medications because the risk to the foetus from the medication is less than the risk of acquiring a congenital infection.

People on anti-malarial medications may still become infected.

Avoid mosquito bites by wearing protective clothing over the arms and legs, using screens on windows, and using insect repellent.

Chapter 11

Conventional Treatment of Malaria

Malaria is a significant problem in India, with potential for severe complications and mortality. Global estimates suggest that almost a million children die of malaria annually, second only to pneumonia and diarrhoea.

It is believed that in endemic areas, some degree of immunity is acquired by the age of seven to ten years, therefore children under five are at the greatest risk. Although strategies for primary prevention such as vector control, personal protection through insecticide coated mosquito nets etc. are useful, they are sometimes not feasible, cumbersome and expensive to implement on a large scale. Since the likelihood of an affordable vaccine in the near future is remote, the use of anti-malarial drugs for prevention could be a useful option, if found to be efficacious and safe. Thus the disease and intervention under consideration are relevant in the Indian context.

Prior to the launch of the National Malaria Control Programme in 1953, malaria was a major problem in India. The disease contributed 75 million cases with 0.8 million deaths every year. After a significant decline in the 1960s, malaria emerged as a major health problem of India in the 1970s. Presently, malaria is a major challenge with 2 to 2.5 million incidences every year.

According to statistical data published by National Malaria Eradication Program, or NMEP, in the year 1997, the incidence of Plasmodium vivax malaria in India was 60-70 per cent, while that of falciparum malaria was 30-45 per cent. Around 50 per cent of complicated malaria cases may lead to mortality if timely treatment is not given, the report says.

As per NMEP survey report (1995), the 'National Average' of falciparum malaria has increased to 35.5 per cent from a meager 9.34 per cent in 1972.

DRUG RESISTANT MALARIA

Drug resistant malaria means malaria caused by a plasmodium resistant to usual anti-malarial drugs. Although chloroquine resistant strains of P. vivax have been described, drug resistance poses a serious clinical problem only with P. falciparum, which accounts for over 70 per cent of cases and much of the mortality of human malaria.

Drug Resistance in India

The incidence of drug resistant malaria is difficult to determine because in many cases it may not be recorded.

Incidence of drug resistance in India is more common with P. falciparum compared to P. vivax. Occasionally, P. vivax may also be drug resistant and this occurs specially as a result of improper treatment and inadequate dosage.

Originally, both the Plasmodia – vivax and falciparum were sensitive to chloroquine, but, in recent years, increasing number of chloroquine drug resistance cases are seen with P. falciparum.

In India, the first confirmed report of chloroquine resistance in P. falciparum was reported in Diphu area of Karbianglong district of Assam in 1973.

To overcome this problem of chloroquine resistance, a sulfadoxine-pyrimethamine combination was used. But, very soon, some strains of falciparum developed resistance to this combination also.

P. falciparum resistances to traditional drugs like quinine have also been reported. In view of these observations National Drug Policy for Malaria has been formulated and implemented with effect from 2007.

Worldwide Incidence

Chloroquine resistant strains of P. falciparum are found now in nearly all areas of chloroquine use including South America, Central America, east of Panama Canal, the Western Pacific, East Asia and many regions of Africa, south of the Sahara.

Resistance to the combination of pyrimethamine and sulfadoxine is prevalent in some areas of Southeast Asia, the Amazon Basin of South America and many foci in Sub-Saharan Africa.

Similarly, variable degrees of decreased responsiveness to quinine and quinidine have been reported, though rarely, in South-East Asia and Oceania and apparently in Sub-Saharan Africa.

Recent reports from Indonesia (Irian Java, Sumatra) and Papua New Guinea indicate high levels of P. vivax schizonts resistant to chloroquine. Resistance of P. vivax blood schizonts to pyrimethamine and sulfadoxine has been reported in many areas of the world, particularly South-East Asia.

The effectiveness of antimalarial drugs differs with different species of the parasite and with different stages of the parasite's life cycle. Your physician will determine the treatment plan most appropriate for your individual condition.

List of common drugs for treatment of malaria:

Chloroquine

Amodiaquine

Antifolate drugs (sulfa drug-pyrimethamine combinations)

Proguanil

Mefloquine

Quinine, quinidine and related alkaloids

Halofantrine

Artemisinin and its derivatives

Primaquine

Antibiotics used as antimalarial drugs

Atovaquone-proguanil

Chloroquine-proguanil

Artemether-lumefantrine

Mefloquine-sulfadoxine-pyrimethamine

These drugs should be taken under proper guidance of the physician, only after the correct diagnosis.

Vaccination

Vaccines for malaria are under development, with no completely effective vaccine yet available.

Chapter 12

Traditional and Complementary Therapies

The proven chemotherapy for malaria as per National Drug Policy is the mainstay and sheet anchor for treatment of malaria. Early diagnosis and prompt treatment avoids delay and saves life. The complementary therapies dealt in this chapter are of historical importance. With the passage of time most of these have become obsolete, but some of these however, are still relevant such as increased intake of fluids, cooling the body with water apart from source reduction to prevent mosquito breeding.

HOMEOPATHY

The treatment plan by homeopathy is as follows:

1. Specific for malaria
2. Symptom based
3. Symptoms of the mind in malarial fever
4. Physical generals
5. Concomitants

6. Prophylaxis
7. Mother tinctures

Specific Remedies for Pathophysiology of Malaria of any Strain

1. **Ledum palustre**: For punctured wounds, for mosquito bites and their effects on the body. 30c, taken 3 times each week, may help to prevent bites.

2. **Arsenicum album**: This essentially is indicated for the related fevers associated with malaria of all forms and strains. High, septic fevers with profuse exhaustion. Cold sweats with fever.

3. **Ceanothus americanus**: This is indicated for the typical enlargement of the spleen seen with malarial cases. This remedy stimulates the spleen to function more efficiently in dealing with the disease.

4. **Chininum arsenicosum**: Treatment for the weariness and prostration seen with malaria as well as the associated fevers.

5. **Chininum sulphuricum**: Treats the periodicity of typical malarial fevers and helps to actually rid the body of the malarial protozoa.

6. **Eupatorium perfoliatum**: It relieves the pain in limbs and muscles that accompanies febrile diseases like malaria.

7. **Malaria nosode**: This remedy is made from the protozoa of malaria itself.

8. **Caladium seguinum 6c** and **Staphysagria 12c** is taken if the patient is prone to be bitten by the mosquitoes.

Symptom Based

Fever with chill: Aconitum napellus, Belladonna, Calcarea carbonica, Chamomilla, Helliborus niger, Ignatia amara, Nitricum acidum, Nux vomica, Rhus toxicodendron, Sulphur.

Fever alternating with chill: Ammonium muriaticum, Arsenicum album, Bryonia alba, China officinalis, Hepar sulphur, Mercurius solubilis, Nux vomica, Rhus toxicodendron.

Intermittent fever: Kali sulphuricum, Ferrum metallicum, Lycopodium, Natrium muriaticum, Psorinum, Pyrogenium, Tarentula, Tuberculinum.

Malaria is transmitted by the parasite known as Plasmodium. It has 4 varieties and these are Plasmodium ovale, Plasmodium vivax, Plasmodium malariae, and Plasmodium falciparum.

The symptoms produced by Plasmodium vivax and Plasmodium ovale appear about 12 to 14 days after infection.

1. The classical onset of fever is preceded by many days of marked weakness and lethargy.
2. Pain in the whole abdomen
3. Chills and sweats
4. Diarrhoea, nausea, and vomiting
5. Headache
6. High fevers
7. Low blood pressure causing dizziness if moving from a lying or sitting position to a standing position.
8. Muscle aches
9. Appetite becomes poor, no desire to take food.

Fever with chill

Aconitum napellus

Cold stage is most marked, cold sweat and icy coldness of the face.

Coldness and heat alternate.

Evening chills soon after going to bed.

Thirst for cold water and restlessness always present.

Dry heat, red face.

Sweat drenching, on parts laid on; this relieves all symptoms.

Belladonna

A high feverish state with comparative absence of toxaemia.

Burning, pungent, steaming heat.

Feet icy cold, superficial blood vessels dilated and distended.

Perspiration dry, only on head.

No thirst with fever.

Calcarea carbonica

Chills at 2 pm, begins internally in stomach region.

Pulse full and frequent, chills and heat.

Partial sweats, night sweats, especially on head, neck and chest.

Sweat all over head in children, so much that the pillow becomes wet.

Ignatia amara

Chill, with thirst; relieved by external heat.

Itching during fever.

Nettle rash all over body.

Nux Vomica

Cold stage predominates.

Excessive rigor, with blueness of finger nails.

Chilly; must be covered in every stage of fever.

Perspiration sour; only on one side of the body.

Chilliness on being uncovered, yet he does not allow being covered.

Dry heat of the body.

Rhus toxicodendron

Intermittent chills, with dry cough and restlessness.

Urticaria during heat.

Chilly as if cold water has been poured over him, followed by heat.

Sulphur

Frequent flashes of heat.

Dry skin and great thirst.

Night sweats on nape and occiput.

Perspiration of single parts.

Remittent type of fever.

Fever Alternating with Chill

Ammonium muriaticum

Chills during the evenings after lying down and on awakening, without thirst.

Palms and soles hot to touch.

Sub acute, low fever due to unhealthy climate.

Arsenicum album

Periodicity marked with adynamia.

Intermittent type of fever.

Paroxysms incomplete with marked exhaustion.

Cold sweat all over body.

Great restlessness mental as well as physical.

Bryonia

Pulse full, hard, tense and quick.

Chills with external coldness, dry cough, stitching character.

Sweat sour after slight exertion.

Sweat is profuse and comes easily.

Thirst for large quantities at longer intervals.

China officinalis

Intermittent paroxysms return every week.

Chills, generally in afternoon.

Thirst before chill, for small quantities at short intervals.

Cocculus indicus

Chill with flatulent colic.

Nausea, vertigo, coldness in the lower extremities.

Nervous form of low fevers.

Chilliness with perspiration and heat of skin.

Hepar sulphur

Chilly in open air.

Dry heat at night.

Profuse sweat; sour, sticky and offensive.

Mercurius solubilis

Fever generally gastric or bilious in nature with profuse nocturnal perspiration.

Heat and shuddering alternately.

Yellow perspiration without relief.

Creeping chilliness, worse in evening.

Nux Vomica

Cold stage predominates.

Excessive rigor, with blueness of finger nails.

Chilly; must be covered in every stage of fever.

Perspiration sour; only on one side of the body.

Chilliness on being uncovered, yet he does not allow being covered.

Dry heat of the body.

Rhus toxicodendron

Intermittent chills, with dry cough and restlessness.

Urticaria during heat.

Chilly as if cold water has been poured over him, followed by heat.

Intermittent Fever

Fever with Chills

Alstonia, ammonium picricum, amylenum nitrosum, apis mellifica, aranea diadema, arsenicum album, camphora monobromata, capsicum, carbo vegetabilis, cedron, chininum arsenicosum, chininum muriaticum, chininum sulphuricum, cinchona officinalis, cornus alternifolia, echinacea, eupatorium perfoliatum, eupatorium purpureum, gelsemium sempervirens, helianthes, ignatia amara, ipecacuanha, lachesis mutus, menyanthes trifoliata, natrium muriaticum, nux vomica, phosphoricum acidum, tela aranearum, veratrum album.

Ferrum metallicum

Generalized coldness of the extremities.

Head and face hot.

Chill at 4 pm.

Heat in palms and soles.

Sweat is profuse and debilitates the patient.

Kalium sulphuricum

Rise of temperature at night.

Tongue during fever is yellow and slimy.

Lycopodium clavatum

Chill between 3 and 4 pm, followed by sweat.

Icy coldness, as if lying on the ice.

One chill is followed by another.

Natrium muriaticum

Chill between 9 and 11 am.

Heat; violent thirst, increases with fever.

Coldness of the body and continuous chilliness.

Sweats on every exertion.

Pyrogenium

Coldness and chilliness.

Septic fevers.

Chill begins in the back.

Temperature rises rapidly.

Great heat with profuse hot sweat.

Chill Every Day (Quotidian)

Aranea diadema, Arsenicum album, Cactus grandiflorus, Ipecacuanha, Natrium muriaticum, Nux vomica, Pulsatilla, chininum sulphuricum, Ignatia amara, Lobelia inflata, Nitricum acidum, Plumbum metallicum, Tarentula hispanica.

Chill Every 2 Days (Tertian)

Aranea diadema, Arsenicum album, Bryonia alba, Capsicum annum, Eupatorium perfoliatum, Eupatorium purpureum, Ipecacuanha, Nux vomica, Pulsatilla nigricans, Calcarea carbonica, Chininum sulphuricum, Cinchona officinalis, Lycopodium clavatum.

Chill Every 72 Hours (Quartan)

Arsenicum album, Arsenicum iodatum, Cimex lectularius, Hyoscyamus niger, Iodium, Lycopodium clavatum, Pulsatilla nigricans, Sabadilla, Veratrum album, Chininum sulphuricum, Cinchona officinalis, Helleborus niger.

Periodicity

Arnica montana, Arsenicum album, Cedron, Chininum sulphuricum

Chill Starts At

Daytime-china officinalis

Morning (6-9 hrs)–Angustura vera, Bovista lycoperdon, Bryonia alba, Conium maculatum, Eupatorium perfoliatum, Natrium muriaticum, Nitricum acidum, Nux vomica, Podophyllum peltatum, Sepia officinalis, Veratrum album.

Forenoon (9-12 hrs)

9 am-Eupatorium perfoliatum

10 am-Natrium muriaticum, Stannum metallicum.

11 am-Cactus grandiflorus, Natrium muriaticum, Nux vomica

Noon-Lobelia inflata, Lycopodium clavatum, Natrium muriaticum, Pulsatilla nigricans.

Noon (12-13 hrs)

12-14 hrs-Arsenicum album.

Afternoon (13-18 hrs)

13 hr-Arsenicum album, Pulsatilla nigricans.

14 hr-Arsenicum album

15 hr-Angustura vera, Antimonium tartaricum, Apis mellifica, Arsenicum album, Chininum sulphuricum, Cedron, Staphysagria, Thuja occidentalis.

16 hr-Apis mellifica

17 hr-Kalium carbonicum, Lycopodium clavatum, Thuja occidentalis.

18 hr-Hepar sulphur, Natrium sulphuricum, Pyrogenium, Rhus toxicodendron.

Symptoms of the Mind in Malaria Fever

1. Anxiety
2. Irritability
3. Comatose
4. Delirium

Physical Generals

1. Thirst during fever.
2. Thirstlessness during fever: Apis mellifica, Cina maritima, Gelsemium sempervirens, Sabadilla, Sepia officinalis.
3. Sweat after the fever: Arsenicum album, Caladium seguinum, China officinalis, Chininum arsenicosum, Chininum sulphuricum, Cuprum metallicum, Ferrum metallicum, Gelsemium sempervirens, Hepar sulphur, Lachesis mutus, Lycopodium clavatum, Natrium sulphuricum, Rhus toxicodendron, Zincum metallicum.
4. If the bites become red hot and inflamed: Apis mellifica.

Complications

Cerebral malaria, which can result in impaired consciousness, seizure, or coma.

Severe anaemia, jaundice, and hypoglycaemia.

Renal failure, including 'Blackwater fever' seen as massive intravascular haemolysis with hemoglobinuria.

Shock (circulatory collapse).

Pulmonary oedema or acute respiratory distress syndrome.

Spontaneous bleeding/disseminated intravascular coagulation.

Prophylaxis

Prophylaxis of malaria

Alternate between Natrium muriaticum and China officinalis, taking one tablet weekly.

In malaria identified zones the prophylactics are:

Arsenicum album, Chininum sulphuricum, Natrium muriaticum Natrium muriaticum 30c once a week during your stay.

Malaria Nosode 30c once a week while away, and once a week for two weeks after leaving the high risk area.

Mother Tinctures

Ceanothus either as a tincture (5 drops in water) or in 6x potency.

Taken daily, this strengthens the spleen and immune system while you're travelling in a malaria risk zone.

HERBAL REMEDIES

Ginger is commonly used for the treatment of malaria.

Take a small piece of ginger and 2-3 teaspoon raisins. Add this to a glass of water and boil it till the constituents become half. Allow it to cool and give to the patient.

Basil or commonly known as tulsi, the leaves are used as treatment for malaria.

Take 12-15 basil leaves and extract its juice. Add 1-2 tablespoon of black pepper powder to it.

Cinnamon and clove powder are used for treating malaria.

Take 2-3 teaspoon of finely powdered cloves and cinnamon and mix in a glass of water. Boil this until the constituents become half. Allow it to cool and add little amount of black pepper or honey to it.

The patient can take this mixture 2-3 times a day.

AYURVEDA

AYURVEDA...Simple translated meaning is 'science or knowledge to increase longevity, means life'.

Life is not merely being but instead 'well being' in respect of body, soul and mind.

Since the time immemorial the sages tried to help society by protecting them from the evils. Morbidity, the ill health was one of them. Therefore, since the ancient times the prevention was also prevalent along with healing. Generally all sages used to learn ayurveda during their learning of meditation so that they be helpful to the society in totality, as they were the most trusted and solvers of all the problems of the common people.

This science was practised verbally, but Muni Ved Vyas preserved the complete knowledge into writing along with ethics, virtue and self enlightenment.

There are two schools of Ayurveda 'Charak' and 'Sushrut'. Charak belonged to Atreya School and the Sushrut to Dhanwantri theories.

The basic theory of Ayurveda is based upon the three disorders or Doshas, i.e. of Air (vayu), of fire (pitta) and of water (kapha).

There are two types of Churans which are helpful in treating the malarial fever.

1. Sitopaladi Churan
2. Sudershan Churan

Sitopaladi Churan

The dosage is ½ teaspoon. with warm water, three times a day for 8 weeks.

The diet in first 10 days is a liquid diet.

Sudershan Churan

This is prepared by mixing 48 herbs. This is taken with cold water.

The herbs which are used in ayurveda for treating malaria are as follows:

1. Amla: This helps in recovering the loss of Vitamin C as a result of high fever of malaria.
2. Neem: This is used internally for malarial fever. It is also used as pills for repelling the mosquitoes.
3. Shikakai: The infusion of the leaves of the tree is used for lowering the fever during malaria.
4. Kutki: The roots of this tree are effective for treating malarial fever.
5. Afsanthin: This can be taken daily to relieve the symptoms of malaria.

Neem

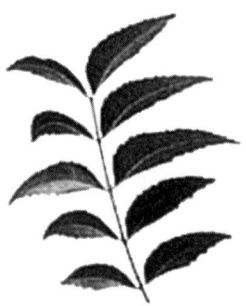

Dosage for treatment of malaria:

Prepare an extract by boiling 30g of Neem leaves in three liters of water for 20 minutes.

Cool it and drink one glass thrice daily till fever subsides.

Ayurvedic remedies for liver complaints:

As malaria is a liver infection the following herbal remedies can also be applied to the treatment of malaria.

Bhunimanala: this is a juice taken from the plant.

Ghritkumari: This is a cactus rich in aloe and other vital revitalizing produce.

All these remedies will help mend the liver and make it more robust to see off the malaria carrying parasites.

Ayurvedic Diet for Malaria

1. A diet of raw or well boiled fruit and vegetables.
2. One should avoid spicy food.

Ayurvedic Yoga as Malaria Remedy

Ayurveda recommends the shoulder stand yoga position to revitalize the liver area. This involves lying on the floor and pushing your legs straight up into the air.

Though like most ayurvedic yoga you should not attempt this without the supervision of a qualified yoga instructor.

Though malaria is an unpreventable misfortune, the ayurvedic philosophy can help you heal your liver properly to help it fight against the spread of the parasites and against further infection.

ACUPUNCTURE

The term Acupuncture is derived from the Latin word called 'acus' means needles and 'pungere' means to puncture or prick. Acupuncture is a pathy where the treatment is done by inserting needles on pre-determined points over the body.

The theory behind this comes from a warrior who during the war got wounded by an arrow and when the arrow was removed the wound healed. And a disease which is not related to the part of wound by an arrow, led to a belief that there is a correlation between the punctured point and the disease it cured. With time various such points were framed and the people of China started the treatment of diseases by putting needles on these points.

The body was divided into meridians thinking that the energy flows through the human body continuously which is called as CHI or Qi. The proper flow of the energy is called as health and if any derangement occurs it is called as disease, which is represented by various signs and symptoms.

And if the 'Qi' flow stops the person dies.

According to the theory of acupuncture there is a constant use and formation of this energy, either in the body through the food which we take and from the atmosphere through the oxygen and water from outside.

The Chinese found that there are certain points on the body surface and when these points were punctured it cured a disease in a particular organ. They joined all these points, and such points were given the name as Meridians.

These Meridians are in two directions, that is, centripetal and centrifugal.

The treatment is done by using various needles of different shapes and metals like gold, silver and stainless steel.

Acupuncture can treat disease as well as the complications caused by malarial fever.

According to the theory of acupuncture the disease occurs due to derangement of the nutrient qi and the defensive qi (Weiqi), which affects the human beings and the disease, is presented as alternate fever and chills.

The main aim of the treatment is to regulate the Du Channel and harmonize the Shaoyang Channels.

Prescription

Dazhui (DU 14.). This is the main point.

Taodao (Du 13.).

Foot-Linqi (G.B. 41.).

Houxi (S.1.3.).

Janshi (P.5.).

For high fever: Quchi (L.1. 11.), needling with the reducing methods.

A mass in the right hypochondrium: Zhangmen (Liv.13.)-Huangmen (U.B.51.).Apply acupuncture at the former point and moxibustion at the latter point.

In severe delirium and mental confusion: Prick the twelve Jing-Well Points of the hand (Lu. 11., H.9., L.1. 1., S.J.1., S.1. 1.).

Treatment is given 1-2 hours before the attack of the malaria fever for continuously three days. Retain needles for one hour.

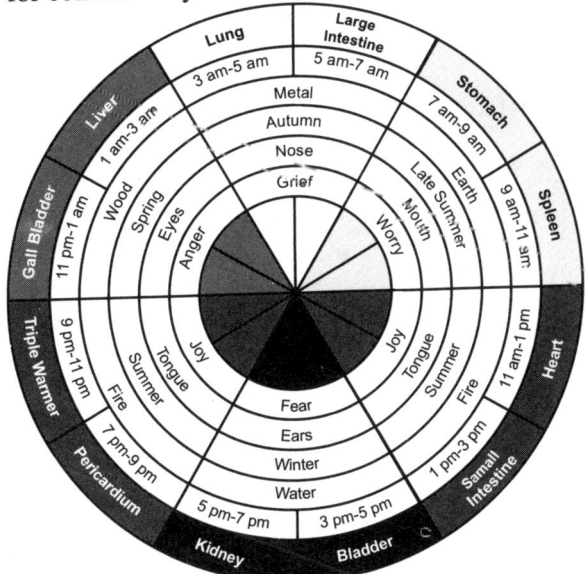

The time frame and the organs involved.

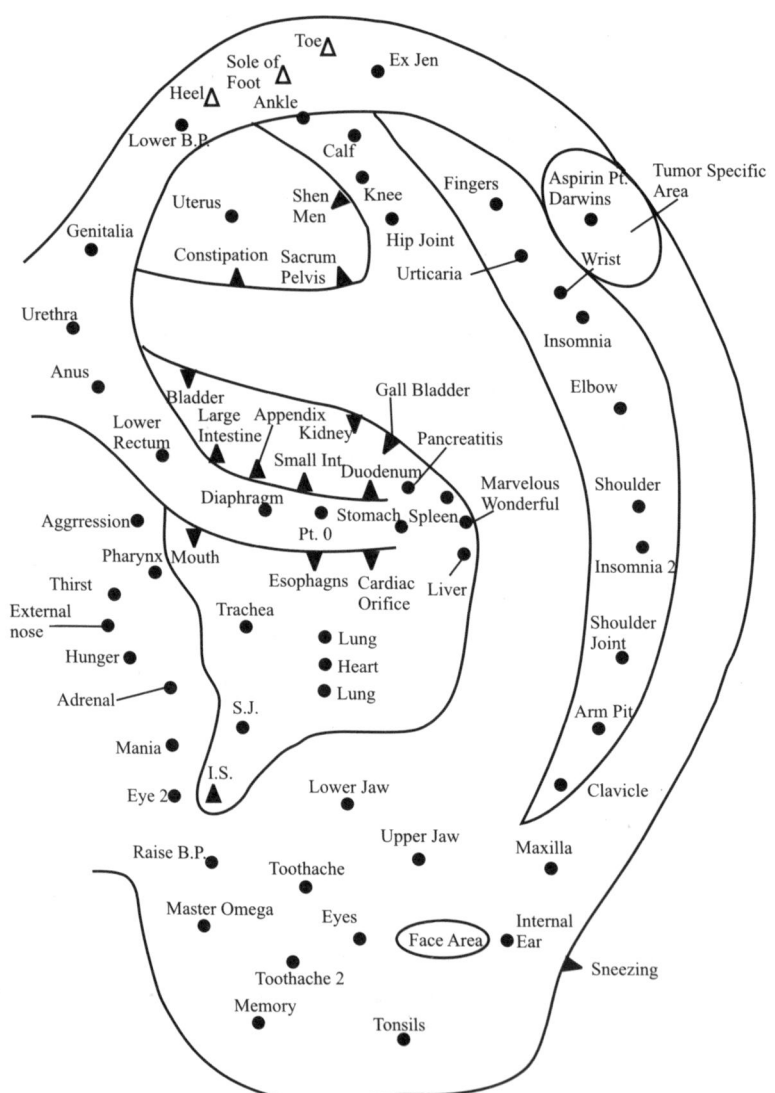

The acupuncture points on the ear.

YOGA AND EXERCISES

Yoga and Meditation

The meaning of Yoga is union of PRAN (inward moving air) and APAN (outward moving air). This means the overpowering of death by life, which is only possible if one has a disciplined way of living.

Yoga teaches self discipline. One becomes master of one's body, mind and soul. By doing exercises regularly one can repel many diseases. The flexibility of your body and mind is in your control. This can be achieved by doing various ASANS (postures). These are further divided into three methods- HATHA, KUNDALINI and ASHTANG ASANS.

With Pranayam, many respiratory tract diseases are cured without the aid of any medicines. Women can deliver babies without feeling any pain.

It is important that you should not force any ASAN against nature. Let yourself feel the completeness gradually. Western world is getting overwhelmed with the achievement of YOGA.

In the treatment of malaria apart from taking the medicines one can strengthen the immune system by doing asans to rejuvenate the liver and the spleen.

The shoulders stand yoga position to revitalize the liver area.

This involves lying on the floor and pushing your legs straight up into the air.

First Step

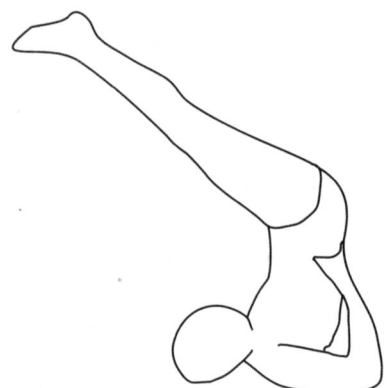

Second Step

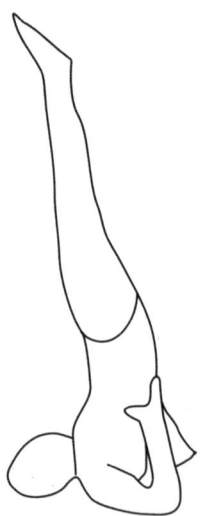

Technique for doing this yoga:

1. Lie flat on your back. Inhale deeply while raising your legs and spine until the toes point to the ceiling.
2. The body rests on the shoulders and the back of the neck. The body is supported by the hands, which are placed on the center of the spine between the waist and the shoulder blades. Keep your spine and legs straight.

3. Breathe slowly and deeply with the abdomen and concentrate on the thyroid gland. On a male, the thyroid gland is located behind the Adam's apple. For women, it is located in the same area which is a few inches above the sternal notch (hollow of the neck where the neck joins the rest of the body.) or approximately half way up the neck from the sternal notch. Stay in this position for about two minutes.
4. To come out of this posture, just bend your knees, curve your back and slowly return to lying on the floor while exhaling. First bend your knees, put the palms on the floor, then curving the spine, gradually unfold it the way one unrolls a carpet. When your entire back touches the floor, straighten the knees, take a deep breath and slowly lower your legs to the ground while breathing out.
5. If you wish, you may go straight into the next posture (the 'reverse posture') instead of lying down.

Time

Retain this position for fifteen seconds to six minutes, adding fifteen seconds per week.

Caution

Do not try this exercise if you are suffering from organic disorders of the thyroid gland. Be very cautious if you are suffering from chronic nasal catarrh.

JUICE THERAPY

Fruit and Vegetable Juice Therapy

The theory behind the fruit and vegetable juice therapy is based upon the recommendations made 2400 years back by the father of medicine, Hippocrates that 'Let living or the natural food be thy medicine'.

In chorus Dr. Stanley Davidson, Dr. John B. Lust, Dr. Louis Kulne, to name a few, had also maintained that our system and blood gets contaminated and there is accumulation of toxins due to the consumption of unnatural and cooked food and hence detoxification is required to rejuvenate the body and system. This in fact is supposed to be the main role of fresh fruits and vegetables. It is like that when there is no garbage in the body the germs will not have any host or media to grow or multiply. Hence the body remains free of diseases. With their version it seems that fruit and vegetable juice therapy acts like a cleansing mechanism as done through dialysis or lavage.

The old saying that *'An apple a day keeps the doctor away'* does not refer to one particular fruit but is a general self explanatory statement regarding the well known importance of fruits and vegetables.

As we are discussing malaria in particular it will not be out of place to mention that the extract of neem is very useful in the treatment of malarial fever. Also many fruits and vegetables revitalize the liver functions which get affected due to malaria.

Other fruits and vegetables useful for malaria are grapefruit, carrot, spinach, celery and parsley.

DIET AND NUTRITION

Let food be your medicines and medicines be your food

Hippocrates

Fast on orange juice and water for a few days. Diet is of utmost importance in the treatment of malaria. To begin with, the patient should fast on orange juice and water for a few days, depending on the severity of the fever.

Fresh fruit Diet

After the fever has subsided, the patient should be placed on an exclusive fresh fruit diet for the first few days. Milk may then be added to the diet.

Well balanced diet, emphasis on fresh fruits, and raw vegetables.

Thereafter, the patient may gradually embark upon a well balanced diet of natural foods, with emphasis on fresh fruits, and raw vegetables.

HOME REMEDIES

Malaria Treatment using grapefruit

Grapefruit is one of the most effective home remedies for malaria. It should be taken daily. It contains a natural quinine like substance which can be extracted from the fruit by boiling a quarter of a grapefruit and straining its pulp.

Malaria Treatment using fever nut

The seeds of the fever nut plant are another effective remedy for malaria. They can be obtained from a herbal store and preserved in a phial for use when required. About six grams of these seeds should be given with a cup of water two hours before the expected onset of the paroxysm of fever, and a second dose should be given one hour after the attack. The paroxysm can thus be avoided but even if it occurs, the same procedure should be resorted to on that day and it will cut short the fever.

Malaria treatment using datura

The leaves of the datura plant are useful in the tertian type of malarial fever. About two and a half freshly sprouted leaves of this plant should be made into a pill by rubbing them with jaggery and administered two hours before the onset of the paroxysm.

Malaria treatment using cinnamon

Cinnamon is regarded as a valuable remedy for malaria. One teaspoonful should be coarsely powdered and boiled in a glass of water with a pinch of pepper powder and honey. This can be used beneficially as a medicine for malaria.

Malaria treatment using chirayata

The herb chirayata, botanically known as swertia andrographis paniculata, is also beneficial in the treatment of intermittent malarial fevers. It helps in lowering the temperature. An infusion of the herb, prepared by steeping 15 gm of chirayata in 250 ml of hot water with aromatics like cloves and cinnamon, should be given in doses of 15 to 30 ml.

Malaria treatment using lime and lemon

Lime and lemon are valuable in the Quartan type of malarial fever. About three grams of lime should be dissolved in about 60 ml of water and the juice of one lemon added to it. This water should be taken before the onset of the fever.

Malaria Treatment using alum

Alum is also useful in malaria. It should be roasted over a hot plate and powdered. Half a teaspoon should be taken about four hours before the expected attack and half a teaspoon every two hours after it. This will give relief.

Malaria Treatment using holy basil

The leaves of holy basil are considered beneficial in the prevention of malaria. An infusion of a few leaves can be taken daily for this purpose. The juice of about eleven grams of leaves of holy basil mixed with three grams of powder of black pepper can be taken beneficially in the cold stage of the malarial fever. This will check the severity of the disease.

MASSAGE

Massage Therapy

The massage therapy is a 'hands-on' therapy where muscles and soft tissues of the body are massaged to improve the health and well being of the patient.

The Chinese medical literature about 4,000 years ago described about the massage therapy. The contemporary form of massage was known as Swedish massage. There are approximately 100 different massage and body work techniques.

Aromatherapy massage: Essential oils from plants are massaged into the skin to enhance the healing and relaxing effects of massage.

Craniosacral massage: Gentle pressure is applied to the head and spine to correct imbalances and restore the flow of cerebrospinal fluid in these areas.

Lymphatic massage: Light, rhythmic strokes are used to improve the flow of lymph

Myofascial release: Gentle pressure and body positioning are used to relax and stretch the muscles, fascia, and related structures.

Polarity therapy: A form of energy healing, polarity therapy stimulates and balances the flow of energy within the body to enhance health and well being.

Rolfing: Pressure is applied to the fascia to stretch it, lengthen it, and make it more flexible. The goal of this technique is to realign the body so that it conserves energy, releases tension, and functions better.

Shiatsu: Gentle finger and hand pressure are applied to specific points on the body to relieve pain and enhance the flow of energy through the body's energy pathways.

Sports massage: Often used on professional athletes and other active individuals, sports massage can enhance performance and prevent and treat sports related injuries.

Swedish massage: Various strokes and pressure techniques are used to enhance the flow of blood to the heart, remove waste products from the tissues, stretch ligaments and tendons, and ease physical and emotional tension.

Trigger point massage: Pressure is applied to 'trigger points' (tender areas where the muscles have been damaged) to alleviate muscle spasms and pain.

NATUROPATHY

Naturopathy and Home Remedies

Naturopathy is the term allocated to the process of healing of morbidity through nature i.e. the healing through natural vegetations e.g. herbs, nutritional diet and the NATURE of an individual. There should be positive vibes in the thought process of the individual to overcome bad health along with the help of other natural resources.

To maintain a healthy life one must also understand the causes as to how certain diseases originate. Therefore, the prevention part becomes of utmost importance as always propagated by WHO. This obviously includes a healthy body, knowledge of right kind of balanced diet through readings of our rich cultural traditions and positivity against any ailment.

The study will take us to the really effective home remedies. It will not be out of place to mention that quality and commercial medicine manufacturing is totally based upon the ancient researches done by our vaids and elders on the naturally available resources like herbs, fruits, vegetables, oils and what not. They knew about the presence of friendly enzymes and alkaloids in these substances. They even knew how a simple superficial bandage (poultice) of soil or some leaves can give instant and miraculous relief. A simple clove acts as a local anaesthetic specially in toothaches. There is an endless list.

They made everything look and prove useful. WHO is advocating only breast feeding till the age of 6 months and the value of ORS (Oral Rehydration Solution). These are nothing but natural and home remedies, which have been culminating since time immemorial. These remedies are easily exercised through the things available in any household at any given point of time.

Hence, in malaria, as I have said, the preventive aspect becomes of utmost importance such as to avoid collection of water near your home which lets the mosquito breed. All the prevention aspects as mentioned should be exercised.

Then to overcome weakness a balanced diet should be given which may rejuvenate the patient as early as possible.

According to naturopathy, however, the real causes of malaria are wrong feeding habits and a faulty style of living, which result in the system being clogged with accumulated systemic refuse and morbid matter. It is on this soil that the malaria germ breeds. The liberal intake of flesh foods, tinned and other denatured foods, and alcoholic beverages lowers the vitality of the system and paves the way for the development of malaria.

Warm water Enema

A warm water enema should be administered daily during the juice and water fast to cleanse the bowels.

Cold Pack Application to the Whole Body

The best way to reduce temperature naturally during the course of the fever is by means of a cold pack, which can be applied to the whole body. This pack is made by wringing out a sheet or any other large square piece of linen material in cold water, wrapping it right round the body and legs of the patient (twice round would be best), and then covering it completely with a small blanket or similar warm material. This pack should be applied every three hours during the day while the temperature is high and kept on for an hour or so. Hot water bottles may be kept on the feet and against the sides of the body.

Prevent mosquito bites, ensure cleanliness of surrounding areas.

AROMA THERAPY

Aroma therapy is the science of treating the person as a whole by using volatile oils. This has been in use since 1000 years. The Persians, Chinese, Egyptians and Greeks have been using the oils of nutmeg, cedar, clove and cinnamon for healing the sicks. Aroma therapy is inhaled through the nose and the oil triggers the senses, which activates the dormant functions of the body.

In malaria, the most common use in aromatherapy is of the cinchona bark. The bark of the cinchona officinalis is dried and softened in wine to make the essence.

Glossary

Anaemia

A decrease in number of red blood cells and/or quantity of haemoglobin. Malaria causes anaemia through rupture of red blood cells. The anaemia caused may be extreme. Pallor may be visible in the patient.

Cerebral Malaria

This grave complication of malaria involves malaria infection of the very small capillaries that flow through the tissues of the brain. This complication has a fatality rate of 15% or more, even when treated and is extremely serious.

Congenital Malaria

Malaria acquired from the mother at birth.

Exit Trap

A trap constructed to capture mosquitoes that are exiting a house or structure. Exit traps are often used in studies that compare the tendency of mosquitoes to rest indoors after feeding versus to those who fly outside after feeding.

Hypnozoite

A stage of malaria parasites found in liver cells. After sporozoites invade liver cells, some develop into latent forms called hypnozoites. They become active months or years later, producing a recurrent malaria attack.

Hypoglycaemia

Blood glucose less than the lower value of normal. Glucose levels of 40 and below constitute severe hypoglycaemia, a life threatening emergency. Hypoglycaemia is common in malaria, as malaria parasitized red blood cells utilize glucose 75 times faster than uninfected cells.

Imported malaria

A case of malaria that is brought into an area by someone who has become infected somewhere else. The person could be either a tourist or immigrant.

Induced malaria

Malaria acquired through artificial means (e.g. blood transfusion, dirty syringes, or malariotherapy).

Introduced malaria

Malaria acquired by mosquito transmission from an imported case in an area where malaria is not a regular occurrence.

Paroxysm

A sudden attack or increase in intensity of a symptom, usually occurring in intervals. Malaria is classically described as producing fever paroxysms; sudden severe temperature elevations accompanied by profuse sweating.

Recrudescense

A repeated attack of malaria (short term relapse or delayed), due to the survival of malaria parasites in red blood cells.

Recurrence

A repeated attack weeks, months, or occasionally years, after initial malaria infection, also called a long term relapse. Due to reinfection of red blood cells from malaria parasites (hypnozoites) that persisted in liver cells (hepatocytes).

Residual treatment

Treatment of houses, animal sheds, and other buildings where people or animals spend night time hours with insecticide that has residual effectiveness.

Splenomegaly

An enlarged spleen. A common finding in malaria patients that sometimes can be detected by physical examination. May occur in otherwise asymptomatic patients and is of use in conducting malaria surveys of a community, although it should not be the only factor considered when counting cases.

Endemic Malaria: Constant incidence over a period of many successive years in an area.

Epidemic Malaria: Periodic or occasional sharp increase of malaria in a given indigenous community.

Stable Malaria: Amount of transmission is high without any marked fluctuation over years though seasonal fluctuations occur.

Unstable Malaria: Amount of transmission changes from year to year.

Vulnerability: Either proximity to malarious areas or liability to frequent influx of infected people or anophele mosquitoes.

Receptivity: Habitual presence of vector anophele mosquitoes or existence of ecological factors.

Clinical Cure: Relief of symptoms without complete elimination of parasites.

Radical Cure: Elimination of parasites actually responsible for attack of malaria.

Recrudescence: Renewed clinical activity seen during the first 8-10 weeks after primary attack (short term relapse).

Recurrence: Renewed clinical activity seen around 30th - 40th week following primary attack (long term relapse)

Clinically Latent: Symptomless phase between primary attack and relapse with splenomegaly, no parasite seen in peripheral smear.

Insecticidal Resistance: Development of resistance i.e. ability in strains of insects to tolerate doses of toxicants which would prove lethal to the majority of the insect population of the same species.

Epidemiological Indices

Annual Blood Examination Rate (A.B.E.R.) = Smears examined in a year x 100 / Total population.

Annual Parasitic Incidence (A.P.I.) = Total no. of positive slides for parasite in a year x 1000 / Total population.

Annual Falciparum Incidence = Total positive PF in a year x 1000 / Total population.

Slide Positivity Rate (S.P.R.) = Total positive x 100 / Total slides examined.

Slide Falciparum Rate (S.F.R.) = Total positive PF x 100 / Slides examined.

P. falciparum Percentage (PF %) = Total positive for P. falciparum x 100 / Total positive for MP

Entomological Parameters

Adult vector density - Man hour hand captures (per man hour density) = No. of mosquitoes collected/ No. of man hours spent in search.

Sporozoite Rate (%) for each species = (No. of positive for sporozoites/ No. dissected) x 100.

Bibliography

1. Akanmori B., et al. Distinct patterns of cytokine regulation in discrete clinical forms of Plasmodium falciparum malaria. Eur Cytokine Netw 2000 Mar;11(1):113-8.
2. Bastos F., et al. Co-infection with malaria and HIV in injecting drug users in Brazil: A new challenge to public health? Addiction 1999 Aug;94(8):1165-74.
3. Bloland P., et al. Maternal HIV infection and infant mortality in Malawi: evidence for increased mortality due to placental malaria infection. AIDS 1995, 9:721-6.
4. Dayachi F., et al. Decreased mortality from malaria in children with symptomatic HIV infection. Int Conf AIDS. 1991 Jun 16-21;7(2):164 (abstract no. W.A.1291).
5. Elm J., et al. Serological cross-reactivities between the retroviruses HIV and HTLV-1 and the malaria parasite Plasmodium falciparum. P N G Med J 1998 Mar;41(1):15-22.
6. Hoffman I., et al. The effect of Plasmodium falciparum malaria on HIV-1 RNA blood plasma concentration. AIDS 1999, 13:487-94.
7. Ittarat W., et al. The effects of quinine and artesunate treatment on plasma tumor necrosis factor levels in malaria-infected

patients. Southeast Asian J Trop Med Public Health 1999 Mar;30(1): 7-10.

8. Kalyesubula I., et al. Effects of malaria infection in human immunodeficiency virus type 1-infected Ugandan children. Pediatr Infect Dis J 1997 Sep;16(9):876-81.

9. Kuritzkes D., et al. Filgrastim prevents severe neutropenia and reduces infective morbidity in patients with advanced HIV infection: results of a randomized, multicenter, controlled trial. AIDS 12(1):65-74, 1998.

10. Mathe C., et al. Potential inhibitors of HIV integrase. Nucleosides Nucleotides 1999 Apr-May;18(4-5):681-2.

11. Okereke C. Management of HIV-infected pregnant patients in malaria-endemic areas: therapeutic and safety considerations in concomitant use of antiretroviral and antimalarial agents. Clin Ther 1999 Sep;21(9):1456-96; discussion 1427-8.

12. Pardridge W., et al. Chloroquine inhibits HIV-1 replication in human peripheral blood lymphocytes. Immunol Lett 1998 Nov;64(1):45-7.

13. Parise M., et al. Efficacy of sulfadoxine-pyrimethamine for prevention of placental malaria in an area of Kenya with a high prevalence of malaria and human immunodeficiency virus infection. Am J Trop Med Hyg 1998 Nov;59(5):813-22.

14. Savarino A., et al. The anti-HIV-1 activity of chloroquine. J Clin Virol 2001 Feb;20(3):131-5.

15. Shulman C., et al. Malaria in pregnancy: its relevance to safe-motherhood programmes. Ann Trop Med Parasitol 1999 Dec;93 Suppl 1:S59-66.

16. Sperber K., et al. Comparison of hydroxychloroquine with zidovudine in asymptomatic patients infected with human

immunodeficiency virus type 1. Clin Ther 1997 Sep-Oct;19(5):913-23.

17. Steketee R., et al. Impairment of a pregnant woman's acquired ability to limit Plasmodium falciparum by infection with human immunodeficiency virus type-1. Am J Trop Med Hyg 1996;55(1 Suppl):42-9.

18. Stoiser B., et al. Serum concentrations of granulocyte-colony stimulating factor in complicated Plasmodium falciparum malaria. Eur Cytokine Netw 2000 Mar;11(1):75-80.

19. Troye-Blomberg M., et al. Immune regulation of protection and pathogenesis in Plasmodium falciparum malaria. Parassitologia 1999 Sep;41(1-3):131-8.

20. Verhoeff F., et al. Increased prevalence of malaria in HIV-infected pregnant women and its implications for malaria control. Trop Med Int Health 1999 Jan;4(1):5-12.

21. White N., et al. Averting a malaria disaster. Lancet 1999; 353: 1965-7.

22. Corbett EL et al, AIDS In Africa III: HIV-1/AIDS and the control of other infectious diseases in Africa. Lancet 2002; 359: 2177-87.

23. www.malariasite.com

24. www.rollbackmalaria.org

25. www.who.int

26. www.wikipedia.org

27. www.cdc.gov

28. http://www.wpro.who.int/sites/rdt

29. www.ayurvedic-medicines.org

30. Repertory of the Homoeopathic Materia Medica by James Tyler Kent.

31. Homœopathic Materia Medica by William Boericke, MD.